NUTRITION
FOR A BETTER LIFE

*"You the individual can do more
for your own health and well-being
than any doctor, any hospital,
any drug, any exotic medical device."*

—The United States Surgeon General, 1979.

NUTRITION
FOR A BETTER LIFE

A Source Book for the Eighties

NAN BRONFEN
Nutritionist for the Pritikin Research Foundation

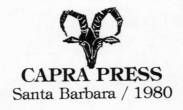

CAPRA PRESS
Santa Barbara / 1980

Acknowledgments:
I am grateful to Nathan Pritikin for the generous use of his
medical library; Josephine Van Schaick for sharing her wealth
of information and resource people; Elizabeth McChristie for
assisting me with research at Reeve's Medical Library; the
many doctors and researchers who cooperated with me in col-
lecting the information contained in this book; Mary Dresser
for typing the manuscript; and my husband for not letting me
rest.

Cover and text design by Terri Wright.

Cover photograph by Wayne McCall.
Illustrations by Alyson Nethery.

Library of Congress Cataloging in Publication Data
Bronfen, Nan, 1935-
    Nutrition for a better life.

    1.   Nutrition. 2.   Health. I.   Title.
QP141.B857   613.2   80-17326
ISBN 0-88496-152-4 (pbk.)

CONTENTS

FOREWORD

Another book on nutrition? There are so many already on the market, with new ones appearing all the time, that people no longer know what to believe. We have been exposed to many conflicting ideas about what constitutes a healthful diet.

It is your responsibility to know how your body works, what kind of nourishment it needs and what happens when it gets the wrong kind. Most of us are ignorant about such matters. We are in the habit of relying on others to take care of us. We depend on physicians to keep us healthy, yet they are trained in the treatment of disease. We rely on government agencies to see to it that only healthful foods are available, but they are subject to pressure groups that do not always have our best interests at heart. We rely on television and the press to keep us informed, but they are inclined to print the sensational rather than the down-to-earth. No one can take care of us as well as we can ourselves. Therefore, we must equip ourselves with the knowledge to do so, and that is why I have written this book—to supply you with the knowledge you need to take care of yourself!

Some of the most popular ideas about nutrition are based on little, if any, research. These books sell well because they proclaim quick and easy answers to problems afflicting man, but they may be dangerous. Sometimes, these books are criticized objectively by the rest of the scientific community, but this criticism usually appears in scientific literature to which lay people are not exposed.

Many popular books recommend diets that are not necessary to follow for good health. Nevertheless some may be more conducive to good health than the diet eaten by many Americans, since they tend to be lower in fat and emphasize fresh fruits and vegetables.

Sometimes, however, ideas in popular books can be dangerous. For instance, certain practices advocated for rapid weight loss have harmful side effects. Low carbohydrate/high protein diets can cause plaques to form on the walls of the arteries. People have even died from extreme weight loss regimens such as the liquid protein diets. Extreme diets have been known to cause the crippling and death of infants and children.

1

These are not meant to be scare tactics. My intention is to encourage moderation and common sense. Be a critical reader. If a book makes emphatic statements, are they supported by facts? Are the concepts tested or did they originate in the mind of the writer? Ideas should be subjected to well-controlled testing. They should not be followed unless you examine them carefully and decide, even though the ideas may not be true, there is little chance of them doing you harm.

This book will tell you about the latest in nutrition research. Putting these findings into practice, will not only increase the chance of greater longevity, but will improve the quality of life. Not only will we be more productive and happy when we are young, but will continue to be in our later years. We will increase the chance of living until our genetically programmed time has run out. We will decrease the chance of suffering from the debilitating and painful symptoms of degenerative disease as we progress from middle to old age.

However, I am not writing a nutritional gospel. Don't accept dogma. That would be dangerous. You must always be open to new ideas. Recognizing the importance of nutrition, more money is being spent for research. Keep abreast of the new advances and although there are many unknowns, act on the basis of what is already known.

Some people believe it is senseless to think about nutrition. "What will be, will be," is their philosophy. They think if they are destined to die of heart disease, it is best not to worry about it. You may have a friend who eats a terrible diet, is a heavy drinker and smoker, and never exercises. Yet he seems happy and healthy. How can nutrition have anything to do with how a person feels?

Perhaps you don't know everything about your friend. Are the stamina and joviality there without being induced by caffeine or alcohol? Can he relax without a few drinks to help him "unwind"? Does his sex life suffer because he eats heavy meals and drinks too much alcohol in the evening? Does he feel good about his body or does he have a beer belly that starts in the middle of his chest? Does he take two steps at a time or does climbing a short flight of stairs cause loss of breath?

Many factors affect how healthy we are. One of these is, of course, heredity. Some people are genetically more resistant to certain things that cause ill health. Perhaps your friend's genetic make-up will protect him—for a while—against these self-inflicted abuses. Perhaps he will live a fairly long life, although it could be even longer. We will never know this with certainty. It is possible your friend would not want to live longer because the years of maltreatment will finally have taken their toll.

We do know with certainty this type of diet and life style will cause a shorter life and the possibility of various diseases in a larger percentage of the population than other more sensible diets. There is always a certain number of people who will be resistant to things that kill others. While improper diet is no guarantee of ill health in middle or old age, it will certainly increase the risk of growing old miserably.

Certain risk factors are statistically identified with many diseases. For instance, the risk factors involved with heart disease include high levels of blood cholesterol, high levels of fats in the blood, heredity, smoking, obesity, lack of exercise, and high blood pressure. The more of these risk factors a person has, the greater the chance of his developing heart disease. This book will tell you how to reduce your risk of various degenerative diseases.

In assuming the responsibility for your own health, you should discuss the risk factors for developing certain diseases with your physician. What *you* know about your risk factors will do you more good than what your doctor knows about them. Know what your blood pressure is. Otherwise how will you know if there is a change in the future? When your doctor orders blood tests, know what the results are and what they mean. If you remain ignorant about the functioning of your own body, you will be less equipped to take proper care of it!

Most diseases are classified either as infectious or degenerative. Infectious disease is caused by invading organisms. Western countries have the technology to prevent many of these diseases by vaccination, and to treat others with antibiotics. Unindustrialized countries do not have this medical technology nor do they have the sanitation we have. Therefore, many of their people die from infectious diseases—especially children under five.

Degenerative diseases are extremely rare in unindustrialized countries but common in Western countries. These diseases include cardiovascular (heart) disease, high blood pressure, cancer, obesity, and diabetes. The best way to prevent degenerative disease is through diet. Except for cancer, diet can often be an effective means of control after the disease has started.

In order to evaluate new ideas you must first have some basic information. I am going to describe some fascinating research so you will understand the rationale behind the diet I advocate. There are many ways to engage in research in human nutrition. Scientifically the best way would be to incarcerate large numbers of men, women, and children and feed them only measured proportions of nutrients, conducting laboratory tests on them, and sacrificing the people at periods to determine the progressive effects of the diets. Obviously, this can't be done so other methods must be used. One method of studying nutrition, is to expose human tissue to certain chemicals in a test tube. Sometimes things occur *in vitro* (in the test tube) as they do *in vivo* (in the body) and sometimes they do not, but from this kind of testing we often gain helpful clues in our nutritional detective work.

Another method employs animal experiments. Bacteria, mice, rats, guinea pigs, rabbits, pigs, and chimpanzees are a few of the animals used. Of course, animals are different from humans; they have different nutritional needs and respond differently to different substances. However, these experiments are not irrelevant to us. Although one could criticize some types of animal experimentation on humanitarian grounds, most are valid from a scientific standpoint. Small animals are often used because they have a short life span. By giving relatively large doses of a substance to a short-lived animal, we get clues as to what might happen with smaller doses in man over his whole lifetime. You may take comfort in the fact that you are quite different from a mouse, but if a mouse dies of cancer after ingesting large amounts of a substance found in a common food, would you want to eat it year after year? If it is clear a substance is toxic to a small animal, it can be withheld from the market until it has been subjected to further testing. It is better to err on the side of caution.

Sometimes small numbers of people are used in human experiments. Although the findings may be provocative, this type of study is usually too small to yield statistically significant results. This means we can never be sure whether the results occurred by chance. It is difficult to control the diets of people unless they are hospitalized. At home, people can cheat or misunderstand the diet. However, working with hospitalized patients usually means the researcher is dealing with sick members of the population. This could lead to many inaccuracies.

The most exciting research compares large groups of people with different diet and health patterns. Epidemiology, the study of the prevalence and cause of certain diseases in different populations, is valuable, although it is hard to control variables. Because they cover large numbers of people, the results are considered fairly reliable.

On the basis of these studies we are becoming more convinced of the correlation between diet and disease. No one study supplies all the answers, but when they are examined together, certain patterns emerge. My conclusions are based on these patterns.

Many popular nutrition books contain numerous case histories and testimonials. While it is interesting to read these cases, they are not scientifically enlightening. Very little is learned from stories of isolated individuals, but much can be learned from the relationship of diet and the incidence of certain disease in large groups of people. Therefore, this book relates epidemiological studies instead of case histories. I won't tell the story of Lucy who came to the doctor's office with falling hair and arches, sour breath and disposition, weakness of mind and body, who was miraculously cured by eating a large amount of a certain food. Instead I will tell the story of an African or American Indian tribe, or a group of Irish brothers who immigrated to Boston, or of the Japanese living in Hawaii. I will show that as the diets of large groups of people change, the incidence of certain diseases changes. When you see the frequency with which these changes occur, the relationship between diet and disease will become clear to you.

Chapter 1

EATING FOR HEALTH

As living beings we must draw our fuel from other living things. We eat to obtain the very substances from which our bodies are made and to provide us with enough energy to sustain life. Energy is necessary for voluntary activity such as mowing lawns, washing dishes, or dancing, and for involuntary reflexes like the beating of the heart and the constriction of the blood vessels. Food is also necessary for the chemical activity constantly taking place in the body cells, such as the repair of body tissues and the elimination of wastes. Energy is required to keep the body in operation even when we sleep and that is why we spend so much time thinking about purchasing, storing, preparing, and eating food.

It is difficult to imagine how the food we eat is converted to energy in our cells. Although this process is not magical, it is complex—and fascinating! This is how it happens.

Food Becomes Energy

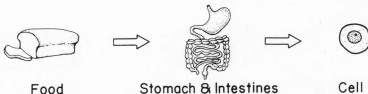

Food	Stomach & Intestines	Cell
· Carbohydrates	Food digested	"Building blocks"
· Lipids (fats)	into "building blocks"	change to energy
· Proteins	· Sugars	(ATP)
	· Fatty Acids	
	· Amino Acids	

Our food is composed mainly of three substances referred to as the large nutrients (as opposed to vitamins and minerals, known as the small nutrients). The large nutrients are carbohydrates, lipids (fats and fat-like substances), and proteins. These large nutrients are composed of smaller units or building blocks. In the stomach and upper part of the small intestine, they are broken down into the constituent building blocks which are then absorbed through the intestinal wall and carried to the cells of the body. This is the simplest part of the complex process. Most of the work is done inside the trillions of cells of the body. In a series of many steps, the building blocks of carbohydrate, lipids, and protein are converted to energy inside the cell. This energy is stored in a chemical form as ATP (adenosine triphosphate). In other words, the energy released from the tearing apart of the food molecules is used to make a molecule of ATP. Later, when the body needs energy, that molecule is torn apart and the energy becomes available to the body.

Energy obtained from food is stored in a chemical form, but is measured in terms of thermal energy: the calorie. In nutrition, a calorie refers to the unit of energy that is potentially available from the food that is eaten. This energy is measured in terms of the heat it could produce. One calorie is the amount of heat required to raise 1g (gram) of water 1 °C. A kilocalorie is 1000 times greater and is the heat it takes to raise 1000g (1 kilogram) of water 1 °C. In the field of nutrition, kilocalories are commonly called calories.

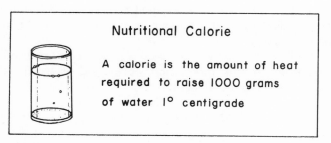

Nutritional Calorie

A calorie is the amount of heat
required to raise 1000 grams
of water 1° centigrade

When we eat more food than needed to meet our energy requirements, the excess is converted to fats. It takes 3500 calories to make a pound of body fat which is stored until the body needs energy and then is broken down producing ATP.

3500 Calories ⟹ 1 lb.
of food   body fat

If our caloric intake is too low, we will die. It can be high enough to sustain life, but still below the optimal amount to maintain us in good health. Conversely, we can get too many calories. About 30% of Americans get more than they need.

Interesting statistics show which members of our population are most likely to suffer the effects of too many calories. For instance, there is a higher incidence of obesity among less educated women. Black women tend to be fatter than white women, and black men thinner than white men. As black people become wealthier, however, the women get thinner and the men fatter. Americans of English, Scotch, or Irish descent are thinner than people of eastern European ancestry. The further east their European ancestry, the heavier they tend to be. There is also a greater prevalence of obesity among members of certain religious groups. The highest incidence is found in Jews, followed by Catholics, Baptists, Methodists, Lutherans, and Episcopalians.

THE DIET OF OUR ANCESTORS

Two scientists, Richard J. Wurtman, M.D., and Judith J. Wurtman, Ph.D., express concern over the rapidity with which our diet has changed in recent years. They have attempted to reconstruct how the diet of our primitive ancestors has evolved to present day.

Dr. Vaughn Bryant, head of the Department of Anthropology at Texas A. & M. University, has been studying the feces of prehistoric man. That's right—he analyzes coprolites—fossilized feces. He finds many different things in his specimens: pollen, bones, feathers and residues of plant material. He then determines the diet of these ancestors of ours. He can also know whether the foods eaten were cooked or raw. He was surprised to find how little the diet of our ancestors changed during thousands of years. He has found evidence that our ancestors ate large amounts of plant foods and ate them either raw or steamed—not boiled. Animals were eaten although they were lean and not readily available. The plants eaten were rich in vitamins, minerals and fiber. Dr. Bryant estimates that fat may have accounted for only 10% of the calories consumed.

Dr. Bryant thinks very highly of the caveman diet and recommends we modify our diet to resemble it. For example, he buys nuts in the shell rather than in the can. He eats many small snacks during the day rather than three large meals. The cavemen found a little food here—a little there—and the "here and there" were often far apart in time and distance. The caveman used no oil since he had no means to extract it. The oils he consumed were contained in the foods he ate, as was the salt. Bryant doesn't use oil or the saltshaker. He steams his vegetables or eats them raw.

I am not advocating the caveman diet. I do, however, want to emphasize that many reputable scientists are becoming alarmed at the ever-increasing rate of radical change in the diet of modern people. While it is not necessary to follow the caveman diet rigidly to be healthy, there is no doubt that it is much healthier than the diet we are presently eating. Remember that man's diet did not change to any great degree for thousands of years. It changed only slightly and so slowly that there was time for the body to evolve and adapt. In just the last thirty years, however, man has made sudden and drastic changes from his traditional

Evolution of the Human Diet

4,000,000 years — Mostly plants; some meat

700,000 years — Cooking begins: mostly plants; some meat

300,000 years — Mostly plants; more meat and fish

10,000 years — Agriculture begins: mostly grains; meat and protein decreases

200 years — Industrialization occurs: protein increases; bulk decreases; salt, fat, cholesterol and calories increase

30 years — Contamination with pollutants and additives; artificial foods introduced diet to one of highly processed, concentrated foods containing many manufactured chemicals.

We can eat many of the same foods the caveman ate but we can learn to prepare them to suit modern taste. These techniques will be presented in a separate chapter. (See *Foods.*)

RELATIONSHIP BETWEEN DIET AND DISEASE

In recent years the relationship between diet and disease has become increasingly clear. We are gaining an understanding of the risk factors in the cause of disease. The treatment of disease used to be the main concern of the health care industry, but because the cost of health care is increasing at an astronomical rate, the federal government is becoming more interested in the prevention of sickness. The Senate Select Committee on Nutrition recently held extensive hearings, including the testimony of nutritionists, physicians, and lay people. The Committee published a report: "Dietary Goals for the United States." Few people are aware of this provocative study. I recommend the first edition because the second edition has changes in response to complaints from food-related pressure groups. It can be purchased for $1.50 from

U.S. Government Printing Office
Washington D.C. 10402

This report recommends that we decrease the amount of salt, sugar, and fat in our diets and that we add more fiber. It says researchers are convinced the changes in our diet that have occurred over the last 50 years are harmful.

Another publication I recommend is *Healthy People, the Surgeon General's Report on Health Promotion and Disease Prevention*, also available from the U.S. Government Printing Office.

EFFECTS OF OVERCONSUMPTION

Degenerative Diseases: Overconsumption of fats, sugar, and refined foods depleted of their natural assets results in many problems. Eating calorie-rich foods has definite esthetic disadvantages. An oversupply of fat is the reason most people are concerned about their caloric intake. However, there are more insidious problems resulting from putting more fuel into the body than it needs. For one, fat people do not live as long as the leaner members of our society. Obesity is related to most of the degenerative diseases. It causes stress to the heart and blood vessels. It causes circulation to slow down and blood pressure to rise. The Senate Select Committee on Nutrition and Human Needs says obesity is a risk factor in cardiovascular disease, hypertension, atherosclerosis, gallbladder disease, and uterine and female kidney cancer. It aggravates arthritis, increases the chance of developing a hernia, and is related to elevated levels of uric acid in the blood. Men between the ages of 35 and 50 will increase their chances of developing heart disease by 30% for each 10 pounds of weight above their ideal. Obesity can cause problems for women during pregnancy and childbirth.

OBESITY

Risk Factor In:	It Also
Cardiovascular Disease	Aggravates Arthritis
Hypertension	Increases Chance of Hernia
Atherosclerosis	Relates to Elevated Uric Acid Level
Gallbladder Disease	Causes Pregnancy and Child-birth
Uterine Cancer	Problems
Female Kidney Cancer	

Longevity: It has long been known that animals, from the most primitive organism all the way to man, live longer when their caloric intake is low. *Tokophrya infusionum* is a one-celled protozoan. Thirty years ago it was discovered that overfeeding causes it to disintegrate, while underfeeding increases its longevity.

Recent experiments demonstrate that the underfeeding of laboratory animals nearly doubles their lifespan. These animals not only live longer but are healthier and less susceptible to degenerative diseases, including tumor formation. It was found the higher the intake of food the heavier the animal and the shorter its lifespan. The most significant contribution to longevity is made when the underfeeding takes place before maturity.

The number of calories a person consumes affects his rate of growth. A negative correlation has been found between growth rate and longevity. In other words, those animals that grow fast are found to live for a shorter period of time.

You may be tempted to overfeed your children, but you will be doing them a great disservice in terms of both longevity and health. Dietary changes later in life will help overcome some of the effects of overfeeding but moderation is even more effective in the young. Malnutrition has been defined as deficiency, excess, or imbalance of nutrients. Accordingly, over-consumption can be seen as a form of malnutrition.

Sex Hormones and Rate of Growth: Several nutritionists have commented on the relationship between the increase in the size of girls in Western countries and their decreasing age of menarche (time of first menstrual flow). The age of menarche has been decreasing during the past century at the rate of four months per decade. Now girls in this country usually begin menstruating at the age of 11 or 12. According to the historian Quarinonius, who wrote in the early 1600s, Austrian peasant girls did not begin to menstruate until they were between the ages of 17 and 20. Today the age of menarche in the girls of two tribes in New

Guinea is between 17 and 18. Heredity is thought to play some role in the age of menarche, and it has been found that girls living at lower elevations begin menstruating earlier than those living at higher elevations. However, the fact that girls of the same genetic backgrounds in industrialized countries are menstruating at an earlier age is thought to be the result of hormonal changes caused by a diet with a greater concentration of calories and by a decrease in their level of physical activity. Accordingly the age of menarche is usually later in female athletes.

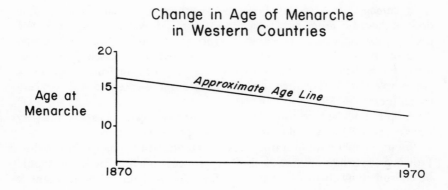

Researchers at Harvard found menarche occurs at a fairly constant weight in girls, and the adolescent growth spurt begins at a relatively constant weight in both boys and girls. Menarche begins when body fat constitutes approximately 17% of the weight in girls. Girls are fatter (relative to the amount of lean body tissue) at menarche than they are prior to that time. There is a minimal weight-per-height necessary for the onset of menstruation, and this occurs earlier in girls who are overnourished. This is why girls with anorexia nervosa (a psychological condition in which they voluntarily starve themselves) stop menstruating and do not start again until they regain the critical proportion of body fat. The same trend in growth and age of sexual maturity is now being observed in countries like Japan where the diet is becoming westernized.

Are these changes good? Does the fact that our children are bigger and mature sexually earlier mean they are healthier and better nourished? Some parents think so but nutritionists do not. Quite the contrary, they see it as a sign of future health problems. Dietary-induced hormonal changes not only decrease the age of menarche but also increase the age of menopause. Both of these factors can increase the risk of developing certain kinds of cancer. Retarding growth and delaying sexual maturity have been found to result in a decreased incidence of degenerative disease and a significant increase in the life span of many species of animals!

A HEALTHFUL DIET

We should approach nutrition with moderation. Too much of any type of food will be harmful and no one food will supply the body with all it needs. It is important to eat a varied diet since no known food contains all the necessary nutrients in adequate amounts. The human body is amazingly intricate. An improper diet will throw off the delicate balance the body tries to maintain.

The diet I recommend will save you money. Spending more for food does not mean your diet is healthful. In fact, costly foods usually do the most damage. As a society becomes wealthier, the health of its people declines because more fats, sugars, and refined foods are consumed. We begin to eat isolated parts extracted from foods, such as oils and sugars. Valuable fiber is extracted from grains and fed to livestock. We eat so many foods deprived of nutrients we have no room for fruits, vegetables, and whole grains. Our digestive systems are not adapted to such concentrated foods.

Simple foods are not only better for our health and cheaper, but they can be delicious and easily prepared once you have learned how.

Some people would rather take vitamins than change their diet. However, vitamins are not foods. They are contained in food, and should be consumed as a part of whole, unrefined foods. Taking vitamins cannot prevent the harm done by consuming too much fat or sugar, or too little fiber. They have no place in the treatment of overconsumption from which so many people in our country suffer. We need not concern ourselves with getting more nutrients but with getting less of the wrong ones.

Some kinds of food—unrefined complex carbohydrates—are preferred by the body as a source of fuel. Americans need to include more of these in their diet. Other kinds of food should be eaten in much smaller quantities. Most foods should come from vegetable or plant sources. They should be whole and only lightly processed. Certain vegetable foods high in fats, such as nuts, should be eaten only occasionally. Foods from animal sources should be minimized as they are also high in fats. Dairy products with the butterfat removed are preferred.

Foods to Eat—Foods to Avoid: Any food in excess can cause nutritional problems, but it is much more difficult to overconsume foods that are high in fiber. High fiber foods are low density (low calorie) foods and are mainly unprocessed plant foods. On the other hand, high density foods are also high in calories. They are extracted foods from which the natural fiber has been removed and in which the calories are much more concentrated. High density foods are high in fats and/or sugar. Sweet foods cause an elevation in blood sugar, followed by a sudden depression and thereby act as an unnatural appetite stimulant.

A DIETARY GUIDE

	What to Eat	What Not to Eat
Dairy	Nonfat milk Nonfat yogurt Nonfat cheeses	Fluid or solid dairy products containing butterfat
Eggs	Whites	Yolks
Fish	Fresh fish(preferable to frozen) Fish canned in water	Fried fish Fish canned in oil
Fruit	Almost all fresh fruit. Limited amount of dried fruit.	Avocados Olives Fruit canned in syrup.
Grains	Whole Barley, Millet Oats, Rice, Rye, Wheat	Refined (white) grains
Legumes	Black beans, Garbanzos, Kidney beans, Lentils, Lima beans, Navy beans, Split peas, Pink beans, Pinto beans, Red beans	Canned beans, Soybeans, peanuts
Meat	Small amounts of lean meat	Fatty meat Processed meat
Nuts	Chestnuts Lychees	All others
Poultry	White meat (Breasts)	Dark meat Skin
Seeds	Caraway Celery	All others
Vegetables	All fresh or lightly cooked vegetables	Canned vegetables
Condiments	Spices Herbs	Sugar Salt

LOW DENSITY FOODS	HIGH DENSITY FOODS
Low in calories	High in calories
High in fiber	Low in fiber
Low in fats & sugars	High in fats & sugars
Unprocessed foods	Highly processed foods

Most high density foods have undergone heavy processing. We should eat foods as they occur naturally, raw or only lightly processed. Moderate cooking—boiling, steaming, baking, microwave cooking—doesn't severely alter the nutritional content of foods. Regard foods in terms of what has been done to them before you buy. For instance, whole grain flour has been lightly processed when the grains were ground to produce the flour. White flour, on the other hand, has undergone heavy processing and has had the bran and germ particles separated from the inner part of the grain.

Eat most fruits and some vegetables raw; cooking destroys some important nutrients. Avoid fruit or vegetable juices. The fiber has been processed out of juices and they are a source of concentrated calories.

Severely limit your consumption of oils and fats. Don't butter your bread or use oil in your salad dressing. Since meats are high in fats and cholesterol, it is wise to cut back on your meat consumption. Always remove all visible fat before you cook meat, skin the poultry, and never eat cold cuts or processed meat.

As you read the chapters on the specific nutrients you will learn more about their composition and their effects on our bodies. You will begin to see the logic behind this diet and understand how you can profoundly affect your health by what you eat, or do not eat.

How much you change your diet will depend on how motivated you are to look and feel better. You may decide to make only simple changes. Or you may want to start out slowly, changing a little at first and making additional changes as you become accustomed to the new way of eating. This approach is often sensible unless a person is very ill, then it is necessary to change more drastically. The important thing is to make a change that you enjoy. The improvement in the way you feel will encourage you to make further changes in the future.

Food and Nutrition Board, National Academy of Sciences-National Research Council
RECOMMENDED DAILY DIETARY ALLOWANCES,[a] Revised 1980
Designed for the maintenance of good nutrition of practically all healthy people in the U.S.A.

	Age (years)	Weight (kg)	Weight (lbs)	Height (cm)	Height (in)	Protein (g)	Fat-Soluble Vitamins: Vitamin A (μg R.E.)[b]	Vitamin D (μg)[c]	Vitamin E (mg α T.E.)[d]	Water-Soluble Vitamins: Vitamin C (mg)	Thiamin (mg)	Riboflavin (mg)	Niacin (mg N.E.)[e]	Vitamin B6 (mg)	Folacin (μg)[f]	Vitamin B12 (μg)	Minerals: Calcium (mg)	Phosphorus (mg)	Magnesium (mg)	Iron (mg)	Zinc (mg)	Iodine (μg)
Infants	0.0-0.5	6	13	60	24	kg × 2.2	420	10	3	35	0.3	0.4	6	0.3	30	0.5[g]	360	240	50	10	3	40
	0.5-1.0	9	20	71	28	kg × 2.0	400	10	4	35	0.5	0.6	8	0.6	45	1.5	540	360	70	15	5	50
Children	1-3	13	29	90	35	23	400	10	5	45	0.7	0.8	9	0.9	100	2.0	800	800	150	15	10	70
	4-6	20	44	112	44	30	500	10	6	45	0.9	1.0	11	1.3	200	2.5	800	800	200	10	10	90
	7-10	28	62	132	52	34	700	10	7	45	1.2	1.4	16	1.6	300	3.0	800	800	250	10	10	120
Males	11-14	45	99	157	62	45	1000	10	8	50	1.4	1.6	18	1.8	400	3.0	1200	1200	350	18	15	150
	15-18	66	145	176	69	56	1000	10	10	60	1.4	1.7	18	2.0	400	3.0	1200	1200	400	18	15	150
	19-22	70	154	177	70	56	1000	7.5	10	60	1.5	1.7	19	2.2	400	3.0	800	800	350	10	15	150
	23-50	70	154	178	70	56	1000	5	10	60	1.4	1.6	18	2.2	400	3.0	800	800	350	10	15	150
	51+	70	154	178	70	56	1000	5	10	60	1.2	1.4	16	2.2	400	3.0	800	800	350	10	15	150
Females	11-14	46	101	157	62	46	800	10	8	50	1.1	1.3	15	1.8	400	3.0	1200	1200	300	18	15	150
	15-18	55	120	163	64	46	800	10	8	60	1.1	1.3	14	2.0	400	3.0	1200	1200	300	18	15	150
	19-22	55	120	163	64	44	800	7.5	8	60	1.1	1.3	14	2.0	400	3.0	800	800	300	18	15	150
	23-50	55	120	163	64	44	800	5	8	60	1.0	1.2	13	2.0	400	3.0	800	800	300	18	15	150
	51+	55	120	163	64	44	800	5	8	60	1.0	1.2	13	2.0	400	3.0	800	800	300	10	15	150
Pregnant						+30	+200	+5	+2	+20	+0.4	+0.3	+2	+0.6	+400	+1.0	+400	+400	+150	h	+5	+25
Lactating						+20	+400	+5	+3	+40	+0.5	+0.5	+5	+0.5	+100	+1.0	+400	+400	+150	h	+10	+50

a   The allowances are intended to provide for individual variations among most normal persons as they live in the United States under usual environmental stresses. Diets should be based on a variety of common foods in order to provide other nutrients for which human requirements have been less well defined. See text for detailed discussion of allowances and of nutrients not tabulated. See Table III (p. 4) for weights and heights by individual year of age. See Table III (p. 4) for suggested average energy intakes.

b   Retinol equivalents. 1 retinol equivalent = 1 μg retinol or 6 μg β-carotene. See text for calculation of vitamin A activity of diets as retinol equivalents.

c   As cholecalciferol. 10 μg cholecalciferol = 400 I.U. vitamin D.

d   α tocopherol equivalents. 1 mg d-α-tocopherol = 1 α T.E. See text for variation in allowances and calculation of vitamin E activity of the diet as α tocopherol equivalents.

e   1 N.E. (niacin equivalent) is equal to 1 mg of niacin or 60 mg of dietary tryptophan.

f   The folacin allowances refer to dietary sources as determined by *Lactobacillus casei* assay after treatment with enzymes ("conjugases") to make polyglutamyl forms of the vitamin available to the test organism.

g   The RDA for vitamin B12 in infants is based on average concentration of the vitamin in human milk. The allowances after weaning are based on energy intake (as recommended by the American Academy of Pediatrics) and consideration of other factors such as intestinal absorption; see text.

h   The increased requirement during pregnancy cannot be met by the iron content of habitual American diets nor by the existing iron stores of many women; therefore the use of 30 - 60 mg of supplemental iron is recommended. Iron needs during lactation are not substantially different from those of nonpregnant women, but continued supplementation of the mother for 2 - 3 months after parturition is advisable in order to replenish stores depleted by pregnancy.

Chapter 2

FOODS

This chapter will teach you how to cook in a more healthful manner, and help you put into practice the new dietary principles of this book. It is not my intention to write a cookbook; however, I include sample recipes to help you get started. The emphasis will be on general methods of food preparation. The chapter is organized alphabetically according to food groups. The different types of food are discussed and a few recipes supplied.

DAIRY PRODUCTS

Milk: There are many good things to be said about milk but it is not a perfect (or even nearly perfect) food. No food contains adequate amounts of all the essential nutrients. Milk is deficient in iron and vitamin C; it is also completely devoid of fiber. There are three main types of milk, differing in fat content: whole milk (3.5% fat), low-fat milk (2% fat), and skim or non-fat milk (0.1% fat). All fat percentages are by weight, not volume. Do not be misled into thinking low-fat milk contains only 2% as much fat as whole milk; actually it contains 60% as much. Remember, milk is mostly water (87%). Fifty percent of the calories of whole milk come from fat and 30% of the calories of low-fat milk come from fat. Skim milk, on the other hand, derives only 2½% of its calories from fat.

For clarification consult the following table.

AMOUNT OF FAT IN MILK Grams of Fat in 8 oz. Glass	
Whole Milk	8.0 g.
"2%" Milk	5.0 g.
Skim Milk	0.5 g.

To avoid fat, use only skim milk, for everyone over the age of two years. Your family may object when you give them skim milk. It is less esthetic because milk has a bluish color when the fat is absent. At first try adding a drop of yellow food color to the milk; it will look richer. You can also mix whole and skim milk until your family becomes accustomed to it. Gradually add less whole milk until you have them "weaned."

In addition to being a high fat food, milk also contains a large amount of sodium and sugar (lactose). Because of the high sugar content, babies should not be put to bed with a bottle of milk. If you feel it's necessary to put an infant to bed with a bottle, use water.

Homogenized milk has been irradiated so that the fat particles contain vitamin D. We require only small amounts of this vitamin and it is made by the body when the skin is exposed to sunlight. Since it is a fat soluble vitamin, it can be stored by the body and we can go for extended periods of time without being in the sun. (See *Vitamins.*)

The fat in milk also contains vitamin A. However, the body can make this vitamin from carotene which is amply supplied in many vegetables such as carrots, sweet potatoes, yellow squash, and leafy green vegetables.

Powdered milk can substitute for fluid milk but fresh milk is better. Heat processed milk powder has had much of the vitamin B6 (pyridoxine) destroyed.

Many people, especially those who do not have western European ancestry, cannot digest the sugar in milk. They have a condition called lactose intolerance or lactase deficiency. Their bodies cannot produce enough lactase, the enzyme that digests milk sugar. Fortunately, the enzyme is now being produced commercially in powder form and can be purchased in health food stores. When the enzyme is added to milk the sugar is predigested.

Milk is a good source of many nutrients including calcium. It also has a good calcium–to–phosphorus ratio which enhances absorption and retention of calcium in the body. Because it lacks fiber and is high in protein and sugar, however, it should be used in moderation. An adult should not drink more than a pint a day. It is not necessary to include milk in the diet because the nutrients it contains are found in many other foods as well.

Cheese: Cheese contains many more calories than milk because it is concentrated. Most cheeses are very high in fat and salt. Processed cheeses have had especially large amounts of salt added.

Hard cheeses like cheddar, jack and Swiss contain very little lactose because it is discarded in the whey. This is not true of the soft cheeses, such as cottage cheese.

Only cheeses made from nonfat milk should be eaten, and they should be used in moderation. You must read the labels very carefully to be sure they are made entirely with skim milk. Dry curd cottage cheese or hoop cheese is always acceptable. If this is not available in your area, regular or low-fat cottage cheese can be put into a colander and rinsed with cold water to wash away the added cream. This works better with the large curd variety.

Cottage cheese used to be made by adding Lactobacillus bacteria to skim milk. Today an acid method is used to curdle the milk. The curds are then separated from the whey and cream is added. Water soluble vitamins are lost along with the whey. Commercial processing also causes a significant loss of calcium. Therefore cottage cheese has a lower calcium-to-phosphorus ratio. For this reason, if a large quantity of cottage cheese is consumed on a regular basis, care should be taken to consume foods that are higher in calcium than phosphorus. Ingesting higher amounts of phosphorus than calcium will cause a loss of minerals from the bones.

We should use moderation and always eat a variety of foods. People are apt to get into a rut and eat the same things day after day. Some dieters are in the habit of eating a cottage cheese salad containing a leaf of low vitamin Iceberg lettuce, a canned peach, and a mound of creamed cottage cheese. Dieters also tend to adhere to high protein diets making the ratio of calcium-to-phosphorus worse.

Many people believe certain types of cheese are lower in fat content than they really are. For this reason, I am including a rather lengthy chart so you can see for yourself you will be ingesting large amounts of fat when you eat most cheeses.

Butter and Margarine: More than 99% of the calories of butter and margarine derive from fats. For this reason, they should be avoided as much as possible. Many margarines start out with completely unsaturated vegetable oils, except those using palm or coconut oil. However, the very process of making margarine saturates (hydrogenates) the oils. (See *Fats and Other Lipids;*) If you must use a spread, try nonfat cheese or mashed banana on your toast. Even a little honey or jam is less harmful than a fatty spread.

Butter, margarine, oil, or other fat is usually used to sauté vegetables in cooking. To avoid their use, you can substitute a little water, stock or wine. If you use fat, you will find you can substantially reduce the amount by cooking at a lower temperature.

FERMENTED DAIRY PRODUCTS
Fermentation is a process used in the production of alcoholic beverages and many other foods, including buttermilk, yogurt, and kefir.

Buttermilk: Buttermilk is the liquid remaining after the fat has been removed from milk by churning. Its food value is almost the same as skim milk but, like yogurt, it contains less lactose. It is difficult to find churned buttermilk any more. Most of the buttermilk found in the market today is

CHEESE
CALORIE, PROTEIN, FAT AND CARBOHYDRATE CONTENT

	CALORIES	PROTEIN		FAT		CARBOHYDRATE	
CHEESE	Total Cals in 1 oz.	Grams / Ounce	Percent of Calories	Grams / Ounce	Percent of Calories	Grams / Ounce	Percent of Calories
BLUE CHEESE	100	6.07	25.9	8.15	71.6	.66	2.5
BRIE	95	5.88	26.4	7.85	72.6	.13	1.0
CAMEMBERT	85	5.61	28.2	6.88	71.1	.13	.7
CHEDDAR	114	7.06	26.4	9.40	72.5	.36	1.1
COTTAGE CHEESE,							
CREAMED	29	3.53	52.0	1.28	38.8	.76	9.2
LOWFAT(2%)	25	3.83	65.4	0.55	19.3	1.03	15.3
LOWFAT(1%)	21	3.50	71.2	0.29	12.2	.77	16.6
DRY CURD	24	4.88	86.8	0.12	4.4	.52	8.8
CREAM CHEESE	99	2.14	9.2	9.89	87.8	.75	3.0
EDAM	101	7.08	29.9	7.88	68.6	.40	1.5
FETA	75	4.03	22.9	6.03	70.7	1.16	6.4
GOUDA	101	7.07	29.9	7.78	67.7	.63	2.4
GRUYERE	117	8.45	30.8	9.17	68.9	.10	.3
LIMBURGER	93	5.68	26.1	7.72	73.0	.14	.9
MONTEREY	106	6.94	28.0	8.58	71.1	.19	.9
MOZARELLA	80	5.51	29.4	6.12	67.2	.63	3.4
MOZARELLA,							
PART SKIM	72	6.88	40.8	4.51	55.1	.78	4.1
MUENSTER	104	6.64	27.3	8.52	72.0	.32	.7
NEUFCHATEL	74	2.82	16.3	6.64	78.9	.83	4.8
PARMESAN, GRATED	129	11.78	39.0	8.51	58.0	1.06	3.0
PARMESAN, HARD	111	10.14	39.0	7.32	58.0	.91	3.0
PROVOLONE	100	7.25	31.0	7.55	66.4	.61	2.6
RICOTTA, WITH							
WHOLE MILK	49	3.19	27.8	3.68	66.0	.86	6.2
RICOTTA, WITH							
PART SKIM MILK	39	3.23	35.4	2.24	50.5	1.46	14.1
ROQUEFORT	105	6.11	24.8	8.69	72.7	.57	2.5
SWISS	107	8.06	32.2	7.78	63.9	.96	3.9
AMERICAN,							
PASTEURIZED							
PROCESS	106	6.28	25.3	8.86	73.5	.45	1.2
SWISS,							
PASTEURIZED							
PROCESS	95	7.01	31.5	7.09	65.6	.60	2.9

SOURCE: USDA Handbook No. 8

cultivated. This means that skim milk is inoculated with a culture of bacteria producing lactic acid from milk sugar. It is the lactic acid that gives it the characteristic tart taste. Churned buttermilk is quite a bit thicker than the old-fashioned cultured buttermilk. Salt and various amounts of butterfat are added to both kinds. This is unfortunate, but you can make your own buttermilk by adding a little vinegar to skim milk. You can drink it, make salad dressing with it or use it in baking bread or fish.

Yogurt: Yogurt is a fermented milk product that has become quite popular lately. It is made by adding different strains of the Lactobacillus bacteria to milk. These bacteria cause part of the lactose to be converted to galactose and glucose, and part to be converted to lactic acid. The lactic acid is responsible for the tartness. The bacteria break down the lactose so they can obtain glucose. For this reason, the sugar content of yogurt is lower than the milk from which it is made.

There are many myths about yogurt. The bacteria with which yogurt is made are believed to enhance longevity, to rid the body of undesirable bacteria, and to have many other wondrous effects. As with so many foods, these claims are greatly exaggerated. Too much yogurt, as is the case with so many foods, can be harmful. Good health is achieved not by eating huge quantities of any one food but by adhering to a diet that is composed of the correct balance of foods.

Yogurt, eaten in moderation, is a good food. It is better tolerated by people with lactase deficiency because the bacteria have digested part of the lactose. However, more of the sugar is digested in homemade than in commercial yogurt. Most of the bacteria in yogurt are killed by our digestive juices. However, to a slight extent, eating yogurt or other dairy products cultured with Lactobacillus will encourage the growth of this type of organism in the intestines. This is not the type of bacteria responsible for the breakdown of the bile acids into toxic substances. (See *Fats and Other Lipids*.)

I especially like to use yogurt in salad dressings. The heat of the oven pilot light in a gas stove is enough to make yogurt. Simply add a tablespoon of yogurt (commercial low-fat yogurt) to a quart of fresh skim milk. Both the milk and the yogurt starter should be as fresh as possible. Place it in the oven before going to bed and in the morning it is finished. To make it turn faster, you can preheat the oven to 250° and turn it off before putting in your inoculated milk. If it has not thickened by morning, remove the bowl, reheat the oven, turn it off and return the bowl to the oven. If you do not have a gas oven you can use an electric one. Heat the milk to 115° before you add the yogurt. Then put it in a warm oven that has been turned off. You will have to remove the yogurt several times and heat the oven until the yogurt thickens. There are many other ways to make yogurt or you can buy a yogurt maker. An article in the April 1980, Sunset magazine, has some good information on homemade yogurt and its uses.

To make salad dressing I add a little lemon juice, onions, chives, garlic, black pepper and whatever spices strike my fancy. Using a lot of chives or green onions makes an attractive dressing.

You can add non-fat yogurt, celery, and onions to water packed tuna to make tuna salad. Bear in mind that a cup of sour cream has 485 calories and a cup of mayonnaise has 1600. Even if you must use commercial low-fat yogurt instead of the homemade non-fat variety, you will only be getting 125 calories per cup. You may not be worried about calories *per se*, but most of the calories in dairy products are from fat and that is something we all need to worry about. They are also high in cholesterol. The lower the amount of fat in dairy products, the lower the cholesterol content will be.

Yogurt can be used in lieu of sour cream on baked potatoes or tostadas. It can be used as a drink, as a dessert with cut up fresh fruit, and in baking. It can also be made into a delicious cold soup. Simply, chop cucumbers, radishes, green onions, and fresh mint and add to the yogurt. A few raisins can also be added. If a thinner soup is desired, add a little water. Season with black pepper.

Never use yogurt made with whole milk, or the sweetened and flavored variety. Make your own with non-fat milk. If you are in a rush you can cheat a little and use the commercial low-fat unflavored yogurt. You will, however, be getting almost as many calories. The low-fat yogurt has 125 calories per cup, the whole milk yogurt contains 150, but the flavored varieties contain about 240.

I am including the following chart to show you the protein, fat and carbohydrate content per 100g (3½ oz.) of regular yogurt, low-fat yogurt and yogurt made with skim milk.

YOGURT
PROTEIN, FAT AND CARBOHYDRATE CONTENT

	CALORIES	PROTEIN		FAT		CARBOHYDRATE	
	Total Calories in 100 Grams	Grams per 100 Grams	Percent of Calories	Grams per 100 Grams	Percent of Calories	Grams per 100 Grams	Percent of Calories
YOGURT, PLAIN	70.	3.94	24.0	3.68	46.2	5.28	29.8
YOGURT, PLAIN LO-FAT	72.	5.95	35.3	1.76	21.5	7.98	43.2
YOGURT, SKIM MILK	63.	6.5	44.1	.2	2.8	8.71	53.5

Kefir: Kefir is made from fermented milk processed not only with lactic acid producing bacteria, but with certain types of yeasts. As with other fermented milk products, the lactose has been broken down so it is more easily tolerated by people with a lactase deficiency. The yeast used in making kefir produces B complex vitamins. Unfortunately, kefir is made with whole milk and contains a large amount of added sweetener.

DAIRY PRODUCTS SUBSTITUTES.

Many people use non-dairy creamers and toppings. These products are often made with coconut or palm oil which are highly saturated fats. Instead of creamers, nonfat milk should be used. If a thick creamer is desired, you can make your own with non-fat powdered milk. Simply use more of the dried milk and less water. Nonfat yogurt is a good substitute for toppings.

EGGS

Each egg yolk contains 2½ times more cholesterol than you should obtain each day. The yolks are also high in fat but the white contains only a trace. In using recipes calling for eggs, omit the yolks and use twice as many whites as the required eggs.

Some people are afraid to eat egg whites because they contain a protein called avidin that binds the B vitamin, biotin, in the intestine, preventing its absorption. This only happens when the egg white is uncooked. Biotin deficiency has been caused in people consuming a huge number of raw egg whites daily or in people on intravenous feeding.

People with heart disease or high cholesterol levels should never eat eggs. One egg yolk contains between 225 and 275 mg. of cholesterol. Dr. Wynder, the cancer expert, recommends no more than 100 mg. a day.

FISH

It is not necessary to include animal protein in your diet. If you choose to, however, one of the best possibilities is fish. Ocean fish is high in calcium, phosphorus, magnesium, iron, iodine, and copper. It contains a high ratio of polyunsaturated to saturated fats, and it is usually lower in total fat than other animal foods. Some fish contain more fat and should be avoided, including herring, mackerel, pompano, bonita and salmon. Those lowest in fat include flounder, haddock, cod, halibut, perch, red snapper, sea bass and sole. Fresh water fish, such as trout and catfish, are more apt to be contaminated due to pollution from industrial wastes or from run-off water containing pesticides. They also contain less iodine and other minerals than salt-water fish. Shellfish, although not particularly high in fat, is high in cholesterol and other sterols, some of which can lead to atherosclerosis. Shellfish, therefore, should be eaten only in limited amounts.

Canned tuna can be eaten if it is water-packed. Never buy tuna canned in oil, and never add salt to it. I like to prepare tuna with mushrooms and serve it with rice as described in the recipe below. I recommend Van Camp's Chicken of the Sea brand tuna because it is packed in cans that do not contain lead solder. Tuna in unsoldered cans contains 1/200 the amount of lead.

Most of the ingredients in the recipes I give are optional and a variety of foods can be substituted for those I call for. You can use more or less of most ingredients, depending on what you have on hand and what you prefer. Remember these recipes are only suggestions to give you ideas. After you get started, you will become creative in the invention of recipes.

Tuna and Mushroom Casserole

½-1 onion or equal amount of shallots, chopped
2 stalks celery with leaves, chopped
¼ lb. mushrooms, sliced
2 cups skim milk
few sprigs parsley or cilantro

¼ cup whole wheat flour
white pepper to taste (I use ¼ tsp.)
6½ oz. can water-packed tuna
4 cups cooked brown rice
1 slice whole wheat bread

Preheat oven to 350°. Sauté onions, celery and mushrooms in 3 tbs. water in saucepan for 10 minutes, stirring occasionally. Keep heat low enough to prevent the vegetables from sticking. While they are sautéing, mix 2 cups skim milk in blender with ¼ cup whole wheat flour, pepper and parsley or cilantro. Add 1 small can water-packed tuna and liquid to saucepan breaking tuna into small pieces. Never add salt, sufficient is added in canning. Add milk mixture to saucepan, turn heat up a little, and stir until it comes to a boil. Put rice in 2 qt. casserole or au gratin dish. Pour tuna mixture over rice. Crumble 1 slice whole wheat bread on top. Sprinkle with garlic powder (not garlic salt). Bake for 20 minutes at 350°. Garnish with parsley.

If you don't want to bake the casserole, simply cook the tuna mixture for a few minutes after it comes to a boil and spoon over the rice.
Serves 4–6.

Ginger Fish

2½ tbs. soy sauce or tamari
3 tbs. cornstarch
2 cups chicken stock or water
2 tbs vinegar
¼ tsp. black pepper (if you do not care for spicy food, use less or omit)
4 green onions

2 tbs. white wine (I prefer pale dry sherry but any dry wine will do)
½ pound fish filet(s), preferably fresh
2 cloves garlic
2–4 thin slices ginger

Mix cornstarch with soy sauce. Add stock, vinegar and pepper. Set aside. Slice white part of onions and cut the green part on the diagonal and set aside. Cut the fish into cubes ½" or smaller and set aside. Press the garlic and finely mince the ginger into a large heavy skillet with 2 tbs. water and saute for two minutes on low heat. Add wine and fish and stir for 2 minutes. Stir cornstarch mixture once more and add. Turn heat to medium-high and stir until mixture boils. Turn off the heat, add the onions. Serve on brown rice with chopsticks.

This recipe contains more sodium than the others. Compensate for this somewhat by serving oranges or other food with high potassium for dessert.
Serves 2.

FRUIT

Fruit is the edible flesh surrounding the seeds of plants. Fruits contain a great deal of sugar and a certain amount of roughage which slows the rate at which they are absorbed. Nevertheless, they should not be eaten in large quantities. Ideally, no more than half a dozen pieces of fruit should be eaten each day, and less of those especially high in sugar such as grapes, plums, and apricots. The high sugar content enables these fruits to be dried, concentrating them. Drying fruit causes the sugar to increase from 15% to 75% by weight. For instance, it takes nearly 5 pounds of grapes to make 1 pound of raisins, and only small amounts should be eaten. Dried fruits are especially bad for the teeth. They are sticky and allow bacteria in the mouth to be exposed to sugar for a long time, especially when they are eaten between meals.

Fresh fruit is full of numerous vitamins and minerals. It is best to eat it raw; many of the fragile nutrients are destroyed by cooking. Sometimes, however, it is nice to have a change. Or perhaps you have a large quantity of fruit on your trees that is threatening to go bad. In this case, simply cut them up and sprinkle with a little lemon juice and cinnamon. Other spices such as cardamom, ginger, curry, allspice, cloves, and nutmeg can be used. Cook them, starting on very low heat, until the juices cook out of the fruit. Add twice the amount of apples or other sweet fruit to rhubarb or cranberries as they contain very little sugar. All fruit, with the exception of avocados and olives, is good for you. Apples, citrus and bananas are the most commonly consumed fruits in this country and I would like to say just a few words about them.

Apples: Apples are an excellent source of pectin, a kind of fiber. This substance is known for its jelling qualities and is used in making preserves. Doctors often recommend apple juice or grated apples to babies with diarrhea. The pectins are also valuable because they cause a very significant reduction in the amount of cholesterol absorbed into the body. Apples taste best when cold; store them in the refrigerator.

Citrus: Citrus fruit is an excellent source of potassium and is very high in the vitamin C complex. The bioflavonoids, part of this complex, are concentrated in the white part of the skin and it is a good idea to eat part of this inner skin when eating grapefruit or orange wedges. Since vitamin C is easily destroyed by air and light, it is best to cut fruit immediately prior to eating. The juiciest grapefruit are the ones that are completely round (rather than pointed at one end) and heavy for their size.

The acids in citrus fruits are corrosive to dental enamel and if large quantities are eaten over a prolonged period of time, it is conducive to the formation of cavities. For this reason, and because the vitamin C in citrus facilitates the absorption of calcium, iron, and other minerals, it is a good habit to eat citrus with meals rather than in between.

Like apples, citrus fruits are especially high in pectin. Strained orange juice, however, contains very little pectin or other constituents of fiber.

Bananas: Bananas, like citrus fruit, contain a large amount of potassium. When bananas are green, they contain 1 to 2% sugar. Fully ripe their vitamin C content is almost doubled, but their sugar content is up to 22%. Consequently it is best to eat green-tipped bananas. If you have bananas you want to ripen, put them in a paper bag. This will allow the ethylene gas they give off to accumulate, and will accelerate the ripening process. Bananas are sensitive to cold and if exposed to temperatures below 55°, they will not ripen properly. In this case they will be a dull, grayish color. In spite of their consistency, bananas are a good source of fiber.

A good way to serve fresh fruit is in salad.

Fruit Salad

3 grapefruit (pink are sweeter), sectioned	Optional:
2 apples, diced	fresh or frozen, unsweetened strawberries
3 bananas, sliced	fresh or frozen blueberries
juice of 1 lemon	melon balls
	pears

Cut grapefruit in half and section into bowl. Squeeze the rinds to get as much juice as possible. Add all other ingredients except frozen fruit. Add frozen fruit 20 minutes before serving.
Serves 4–5.

GRAINS

Grains are the edible seeds of cereal grasses. Most of the calories, carbohydrate, fat, protein and fiber in our diet should come from them. You should eat a wide variety of grains. Gradually begin experimenting with them. In some metropolitan areas many different whole grains are available, but in some places you will only find them in health food stores.

In America, most grains have been highly refined. We use wheat more than any other grain: in bread, cereals, baking, and food processing. In the latter part of the nineteenth century steel rolling mills replaced the old stone grinding wheels previously used to turn wheat into flour. We now use wheat flour from which 28% of the kernel is removed. This processing depletes the flour of its natural fiber, vitamins, and minerals.

Whole (unground) grains can be kept for relatively long periods if stored in a cool dry place. Do not store them near the stove, a heating duct, or over the refrigerator. Whole grains keep longer because the tough outer coat (the bran layers) protect the oils in the germ from exposure to the air preventing rancidity. Flour, however, should be stored in tightly sealed containers, such as those made of plastic, and kept either in the refrigerator or freezer. I keep mine in the freezer. Once you use up the expensive, fatty foods in your freezer, there will be ample space to store your flour.

The best thing to eat for breakfast is hot, whole grain cereal. You can cook it with chopped apples, a *few* raisins or any other fruit. Add skim milk. It is also good sprinkled with cinnamon. Cooked oats make a delicious breakfast. Do not buy the quick cooking flakes as they contain fewer nutrients. Try steel cut oats. They take longer to cook but the taste and texture are better. If you do not care for hot cereal or do not have time in the morning to prepare it, eat a hot bowl of leftover soup, bread and fruit, or leftover salad.

Breadmaking can be a very creative and rewarding experience. Once you get the knack of it, you can use different combinations of grains and a variety of ingredients such as raisins, apples, onions, garlic or poppy, caraway and other seeds. You can try spices such as cinnamon and cardamom, or herbs such as dill, thyme or rosemary. Throw in the cereal left over from breakfast. However, the only essential ingredients of a good loaf of bread are flour, yeast, and water. I am going to give you one recipe to get started but it includes several optional ingredients to show you how to modify the basic recipe.

Basic Bread

6½–7 cups whole wheat flour
3 cups water
1 tbs. or 1 package yeast
1 tbs. honey (optional)

⅓ cup dried minced onions (optional)
2 tbs. tamari (optional)
2 tbs. caraway seeds (optional)

Remove flour and yeast from refrigerator an hour before starting and have all ingredients at room temperature. In a large bowl dissolve the honey in luke warm water. Sprinkle yeast on the water. Add onions, caraway seeds, tamari, and 6 cups of flour. Turn out dough onto floured countertop. Knead for 5 minutes and return to bowl. Cover with a tea towel and a plastic bag and put in a warm place. When dough doubles its size, knead again for a few minutes adding more flour when it gets sticky. Divide the dough and shape into 2 ovals. Put them into bread pans to which a liberal coating of non-stick vegetable spray has been applied. Drape with towel and plastic and place in a warm place until the dough doubles in size. Preheat the oven to 375° and bake for 45 minutes. Remove from the pans and cool on a rack. The cooler the bread, the easier it will be to slice. This bread is good sliced thin and toasted. For variety, try making rolls instead of loaves.

Various conditions—high altitude or extremes in humidity—may call for slight alterations in the recipe. If you should encounter any problems, contact the home economist at your local county cooperative extention office. He is there to help you with problems of this kind.

Remember that more is not always better. This applies not only to the amount of nutrients you put into your body but to the amount of yeast you use when baking bread. Too much yeast will cause the bread to rise too quickly and the air spaces in the bread will be too large. If you make half the recipe for bread, use a little more than half the amount of yeast. If you double the recipe, use a little less than twice the amount.

I specify putting the dough in a warm spot to rise because most people are in a hurry. Actually, however, the bread will be better if it rises more slowly.
Makes 2 loaves.

Spaghetti with Tomato Sauce

whole wheat spaghetti (1 to 2 lbs.)
2–28 oz. cans tomatoes
2 small cans or 1 large can tomato sauce
1 onion, chopped
3 cloves garlic, pressed
2 stalks celery, diced with the leaves
few sprigs parsley or cilantro

¼–1 tsp. black pepper (optional, amount varies depending on how spicy you like things)
1 tsp. oregano and/or other Italian spices *or* one of a combination of the following: minced jalapeno peppers, Ortega green chilies or crushed dry chili peppers

Cut the tomatoes into small pieces or put them in the blender for a couple of seconds. Never add salt to recipes that call for canned tomatoes, as salt is added to the tomatoes during canning. Empty into a large saucepan. Add the tomato paste, chopped onion, celery and parsley or cilantro, and Italian spices. Or you can spice up the sauce by using some of the hotter condiments.

Let the sauce cook for 1 or more hours, depending on how thick a sauce you like. When you are almost ready to eat, start cooking the spaghetti. If desired, add whatever vegetables you like to the sauce—zucchini, cauliflower, peas, etc. The leftover sauce is delicious over rice.
Serves 4–6.

Barley: Barley is an excellent food, high in nutrients and lower in fat than other grains. In addition it lowers blood cholesterol. Unfortunately, it is mainly used in this country in beer and in the manufacture of the sugar maltose. Frequently you will see malted barley listed as one of the ingredients in ready-to-eat breakfast cereals. This hides the fact that sugar has been added.

Pearled barley has had the outer husk and part of the bran removed. Two types are available—light, which is more highly refined and Pot or Scotch barley. Try to obtain the latter. It is delicious in vegetable soups.

Buckwheat: Buckwheat is not a true grain but a fruit. It contains more protein than grains, and generous amounts of the amino acid lysine in which other grains tend to be low. It doesn't have the bran layers that grains do, but is covered by a hull. The hulled fruits are called groats. They are consumed in our country mainly in the form of buckwheat honey and buckwheat pancakes. In Eastern Europe, buckwheat is eaten in the form of kasha, the roasted groats.

Buckwheat groats can be cooked in water and eaten as a breakfast cereal, served with steamed vegetables or with spaghetti sauce or chicken stew.

Corn: Corn is a good food if consumed with other grains and legumes. In societies where corn is the main food, large numbers of the population usually suffer from deficiencies of niacin since the niacin in corn cannot be utilized by the body. For this reason, pellagra is common in places where corn supplies the bulk of the caloric intake.

In Mexico and South America this disease is rarely seen since the corn is treated with lime. You will notice on corn tortilla packages that the ingredients are corn, water and lime. The lime makes the niacin in corn more readily available and increases the calcium tenfold.

Stone-ground cornmeal is usually made of whole corn that has not been kiln dried. Granulated cornmeal has been kiln-dried and milled between rollers. A good deal of heat is generated in the process, destroying many nutrients. It is then sifted and can be obtained in any texture, from flour to a coarse texture resembling the stone-ground cornmeal.

Corn tortillas can be baked in the oven. Do not use flour tortillas; they are made with lard or shortening. To make tostadas serve crispy tortillas with separate dishes of hot beans, brown rice, shredded lettuce, tomatoes, chilies, onions, yogurt, and taco sauce. Let everyone make their own at the table.

Oats: Oats are higher in fat content than other grains. They are also high in water soluble gums which bind cholesterol in the intestine, preventing its absorption. They have been found to be quite effective in lowering the amount of cholesterol in the blood.

We usually eat rolled oats or oatmeal. Steel cut oats, however, taste better. Rolled oats can be used in making bread. Or you can make oat flour by putting the flakes in your blender for a minute or so. This flour can also be used as a thickening agent in place of wheat flour.

Rice: Brown rice should be a staple in your diet. It is an excellent food, low in fat and rich in vitamins and minerals. You will notice that I use it in several recipes in this chapter. If you have to use white rice, choose "converted." It undergoes a process of parboiling and drying before milling. This causes the thiamin and other B vitamins to be driven into the endosperm so fewer vitamins are lost when the bran is removed.

Sometimes white rice is coated with glucose to give it a glossy appearance. In Japan, talc used to be used for this purpose and was thought to be a factor in the increased incidence of stomach cancer in that country. The use of talc is no longer permitted.

Rye: In fertile soil, rye grass grows to a height of 7 to 8 feet. Rye and wheat are the only grains that can be used by themselves in the making of bread. Wheat is better for this purpose, as the protein in rye is less elastic and makes a bread that is heavier.

Pumpernickel is whole rye flour. The whole grain flour is dark, but light and medium flour are also available. Commercial "pumpernickel" bread is often made with the light rye flour but it's made to look darker by the addition of caramel color or molasses. Home bakers sometimes attain the dark color by adding instant coffee or coffee substitutes. You should always choose the flour that is the most lightly processed; that is, the darker flour.

Triticale: You may be seeing Triticale in the markets soon. It is a combination of wheat (*Triticum*) and rye (*Secale*) which have been interbred to produce a new strain. This grain has a high protein content.

Wheat: Many different varieties of wheat are grown in the United States. We use more hard, red, winter wheat than any other kind. Winter wheat is planted in the fall. Spring wheat is usually planted in the spring, but in mild climates it can also be planted in the fall.

The hard wheats are grown in drier areas. The best bread is made from wheat that is 12.5% protein. Hard, red wheats contain 11 to 15% protein and the type of gluten best for breadmaking. Consequently they are used commercially for this purpose.

The soft wheats are grown in more humid areas. They contain 8 to 10% protein and are used in making cakes, cookies, crackers, and pastry. Flour from this kind of wheat is sold for home use. If you can find it, bake bread with hard wheat flour. It is available in some stores and states on the label it is meant for bread baking. Whatever variety you use, make sure the flour is made from the whole grain. Whole wheat flour is also referred to as graham flour.

Macaroni, spaghetti, and other pasta products are made from durum wheat semolina. Semolina flour refers to the large particles remaining after sifting out fine white flour.

Do not use extracted wheat germ. Wheat germ contains large amounts of many valuable nutrients, but it adds substantially to your fat intake and is extremely susceptible to rancidity. Some commercial wheat germ is already rancid at the time of purchase. Even if fresh when you buy it, it will deteriorate rapidly unless stored in a tightly sealed container in the refrigerator.

Bulgur is not an exotic type of grain. It is made from wheat berries from which only the outermost tough bran layer has been removed. The berries are soaked in hot water and then dried until most of the moisture is removed. Then it is cracked into smaller pieces. Because it has been precooked, it can be used after soaking in hot water. It offers a nice change from rice or pasta.

LEGUMES

Legumes are the edible seeds of plants and are contained in pods. They are a rich source of proteins and are especially high in lysine, the amino acid in which grains tend to be low. They also have many valuable vitamins and minerals and are an excellent source of fiber.

Beans: Some legumes require overnight soaking before cooking. Garbanzos, also called chick peas, fall into this category. My family especially likes a soup I prepare using them.

Garbanzo Bean Soup

1 lb. garbanzo beans
1 qt. water for soaking
1 qt. water or broth
1 tbs. finely minced fresh mint
   or ½ tsp. dry mint flakes

1½ tbs. finely minced fresh parsley,
   or ¾ tsp. dry parsley flakes
2-3 cloves garlic, pressed

Soak garbanzos in 1 qt. water overnight, or for 8 hours. Cook them in soaking water, and 1 qt. more water or broth. This takes about 3 hours. Puree most of the garbanzos in the blender with mint, parsley, and garlic. Pour back into cooking pot. Add water or stock as necessary to obtain desired consistency. Heat and serve.

If you enjoy garbanzos in your salad, cook extra for this purpose. *Serves 6–8*.

Chili Beans

1 cup pinto beans	1 tbs. chili powder
1 qt. water	¼ tsp. coriander
3 cups water	1 tsp. oregano
1 large onion, chopped	¼ tsp. nutmeg
2 cloves garlic, pressed	1 can tomatoes (16 oz.)

Soak beans overnight or longer in 1 qt. water. Simmer for half an hour and drain. Cook for 3 hours in 3 cups water. Add onion, garlic, spices and tomatoes. Cut tomatoes into chunks and cook until the onions are tender. Serve on brown rice with a large salad and corn tortillas which have been heated in the oven at 300° until crispy.
Serves 4–6.

Split Peas and Lentils: Neither split peas nor lentils require pre-soaking. I like a spicy soup made from these two legumes. If you do not care for hot seasoning, make the appropriate adjustments in the amount of condiments used in the following recipe.

Split Pea and Lentil Soup

¾ cup lentils
1 cup split peas
2 qt. water
1 cup each onion, carrots and
   celery with leaves, coarsely
   chopped
2 cloves garlic, pressed

1 tbs. parsley, chopped
½ tsp. each coriander and cumin
¼ tsp. each turmeric, marjoram
   and black pepper (or less)
1 cup whole wheat spaghetti
   broken into small pieces or any
   other whole grain pasta.

Wash the peas and lentils in a colander. Add to water in 4 qt. pot. Bring to boil, cover and simmer 45 minutes. Add remaining ingredients except spaghetti. Bring to boil. Add spaghetti. Simmer 15 minutes. Serve.
Serves 5.

Peas: Usually it is best to eat vegetables fresh. When it comes to peas, though, I buy the frozen ones because the best tasting peas are the smallest ones; they contain less starch and more sugar. They are delicious and can be added right from the package to a salad without cooking or defrosting. The fresh peas available in American markets are big, starchy and tough. They are fine for soups and stews but are definitely not a delicacy when eaten uncooked.

The only time I use fresh peas in the pod is when I want to serve them as a finger food. They are nice to serve in a basket in lieu of salted nuts. They are fun to eat straight from the pod and will keep fingers busy so they will not be tempted to reach for greasier and sweeter treats.

Peanuts: Peanuts are really legumes. They are, however, similar to nuts in fat content. Seventy percent of the calories are from fat.

Peanuts should be avoided for another reason, too. The fungus, *Aspergillus flavus,* infests many food plants but it grows most readily on peanuts. This mold produces an aflatoxin which is a potent agent in causing liver cancer. Peanuts with amounts of toxin exceeding limits established by the government are no longer permitted in the manufacture of peanut butter, but there is no way to eliminate aflatoxin completely from peanut products. When aflatoxins are ingested by lactating animals they occur in the milk. It is possible the consumption of milk containing aflatoxin poses a threat to infants. Poisoning has occurred in ducks, turkeys, dogs and other animals whose foods contained peanut meal. Autopsy evidence of liver damage was seen in malnourished children in India who consumed peanut protein powder.

Some molds don't produce any kinds of toxins. The molds that produce aflatoxins are usually a yellowish color. Grains, bread, nuts and legumes should be thrown away if they have any mold at all on them, as should soft cheeses such as ricotta, cottage or cream cheese. If mold grows on jams or jellies made from low-acid fruits such as apricots, pears, figs, and persimmons, they should be discarded. If mold is found on pickled or canned fruits or vegetables, they should be considered unsafe. Some foods can be eaten after mold is scraped away. These include jams and jellies made with acid fruits (all fruits except those mentioned above), cured meats (bacon and ham), fresh fruit or dried fruit, meat or fish. If you are in doubt, throw the food away since the poisons produced by certain molds can be extremely toxic. In California, dogs go into convulsions 20 to 30 minutes after eating moldy walnuts from the ground.

No brand of peanut butter has been found free of aflatoxin. Peanut butter is naturally high in vegetable oils. In addition, sugar, salt, and hydrogenated (saturated) or partially hydrogenated oils have been added to many brands. Partially hydrogenated fats are especially bad for you. (See *Fats and Other Lipids.*)

Soybeans: Soybeans are high in fat. They should be avoided or used sparingly. Tofu or soybean curd, which is used frequently in Chinese cooking, has had some of the fat removed in the processing. Like meat, fish or chicken, it can be used as a condiment in dishes such as Stir "Fry" Vegetables or Ginger Fish.

I am including the chart below to show you the amount of fat contained in soybeans and peanuts compared with the amount in other legumes.

LEGUMES:
CALORIES, PROTEIN, FAT AND CARBOHYDRATE IN LEGUMES AS EATEN

LEGUME	CALORIES Total Calories in 100 Grams	PROTEIN Grams per 100 Grams	Percent of Calories	FAT Grams per 100 Grams	Percent of Calories	CARBOHYDRATE Grams per 100 Grams	Percent of Calories
BLACKEYE PEAS (COWPEAS)	76	5.1	23.3	0.3	3.3	13.8	73.4
LENTILS	106	7.8	25.5	Trace	–	19.3	74.5
LIMA BEANS	138	8.2	20.6	0.6	3.6	25.6	75.8
PEANUTS	582	26.2	15.6	48.7	70.0	20.6	14.4
PEAS (SPLIT)	115	8.0	24.1	0.3	2.2	20.8	73.7
RED BEANS	118	7.8	22.9	0.5	3.5	21.4	73.6
SOYBEANS	118	9.8	28.8	5.1	36.2	10.1	35.0
SOYBEAN CURD (TOFU)	72	7.8	37.6	4.2	48.8	2.4	13.6
WHITE BEANS	118	7.8	22.9	0.6	4.3	21.2	72.8

Carob: Carob comes from a leguminous tree native to the Mediterranean. Unlike other legumes, the pod rather than the seed is eaten. The pods are ground into a powder and used as a substitute for chocolate.

Carob powder is high in fiber and has an excellent calcium-to-phosphorus ratio. It contains a large amount of natural sugar and should be used without additional sweetening. The powder can be mixed with milk, yogurt or water to make a paste to cover pieces of banana. The pieces can then be laid on foil or waxed paper and placed in the freezer. This is a compromise dessert which tastes very good.

Unlike carob, cocoa and chocolate have an unfavorable calcium-to-phosphorus ratio. They contain substances to which many people are allergic and a stimulant, theobromine. They are also extremely high in fat. Pods 6 to 14 inches long and 2 to 5 inches in diameter grow on cocoa trees. It is the beans inside and not the pods that are eaten. Ground cocoa beans are 50% vegetable fat, cocoa butter. A large portion of this fat is removed in making cocoa powder. In making chocolate, however, cocoa butter is re-added. The following chart will give you an idea of the relative amount of calories and fat in carob, cocoa powders and chocolate.

CALORIES AND FAT IN 100 GRAMS (3½ OUNCES)
OF CAROB, COCOA AND CHOCOLATE

	Calories	Grams of Fat	Percent of Calories From Fat
Carob Powder	180	1.4	6.5
Chocolate (bitter or baking)	505	53.0	87.8
Cocoa Powder	347	2.0	4.8

MEAT

Although meat is considered a protein food, approximately half its calories are from protein and half from fat. The calories from pork and lamb are divided about equally, but lean, cooked hamburger contains more fat calories than protein calories.

Until recently meat has been contaminated with DES (diethylstilbestrol). This is a synthetic hormone with estrogenic properties, given to cattle in the U.S. for the past twenty-five years because it stimulates growth. Those fed the hormone also require less feed.

Laboratory animals fed DES develop a 50% higher incidence of mammary (breast) tumors. Many daughters of women who took DES during pregnancy developed vaginal cancer. Some of the sons of these women have been found to be less aggressive, athletic, assertive, and in other ways less masculine than normal males. A recent study shows that in 65% of these men there was history of cryptorchidism (failure of descent of the testes), testicular cysts, a high incidence of semen abnormalities, and testes below normal in size. DES and other contaminants are more concentrated in the livers of animals. For this reason, pregnant women have been advised against eating liver, especially during the first few months of pregnancy.

The Food and Drug Administration has finally been successful in banning the use of DES. However, it is still turning up in meat, presumably from illegal use. There are 143 other drugs and pesticides which leave residues in meat. Forty-two are suspected of causing cancer, 20 of causing birth defects and 6 of causing mutations. Mutations are changes that occur in the genetic material of the cell and are perpetuated when the cell divides. They are the direct cause of cancer. Government estimates indicate that 14% (by dressed weight) of the meat and poultry sampled by the Department of Agriculture between 1974 and 1976 contained potentially harmful residues of drugs, pesticides, and other contaminants. A report to the Congress further states the amounts of these residues often exceed established tolerances. Since the Agriculture Department does not test for most drugs and pesticides that are apt to leave residues, the incidence of illegal residues was probably much higher.

Antibiotics are routinely administered to cattle, swine, and poultry because they stimulate growth and significantly improve feed efficiency.

They also prevent infective diseases in animals raised in crowded and unsanitary conditions. In 1970, 1300 tons of antibiotics were fed to animals in the United States. These dosages aren't sufficient to kill all the infective bacteria. Rather they let resistant strains evolve. In tests, 30% of cooked sausage contained antibiotic-resistant E. coli bacteria which are a common cause of infection. E. coli are capable of transferring their antibiotic-resistance to salmonella bacteria, the organism responsible for food poisoning.

Bacteria in the intestinal tract of man can become resistant to antibiotics when they are exposed to residues in meat. Penicillin, the tetracyclines and most of the antibiotics used for man are also used in animal feeds. Should a person require antibiotic treatment, it is possible that these drugs would no longer be effective. Until 1955, it was very rare to encounter antibiotic-resistant strains of bacteria. By 1965, they were common.

Not all of the harmful substances in meat are put there by man. Malonaldehyde is a breakdown product which begins to form as soon as the animal is slaughtered. It has been known for a long time that malonaldehyde was present in meat, and the amount was measured to find out how old meat was. However, five years ago, it was discovered it is a potent carcinogen. The highest levels were found in beef. Populations who eat large quantities of beef have a higher incidence of bowel cancer. Higher levels of malonaldehyde are found: (1) in beef that is old, (2) in beef that has been thawed at room temperature, and (3) in leftover meat unrefrigerated for long periods of time.

In addition to the undesirable substances in raw meat, mutagenic substances are formed when meat is cooked. They are also in stock. They are found in the highest amounts in beef that has been cooked at high temperatures and in beef stock that has been boiled down and condensed to form an extract for bouillon. They are even present in meat that is cooked at low temperatures.

People who must severely restrict their intake of sodium will have to limit their intake of beef, poultry, and fish as they contain large amounts of this mineral.

Meat and poultry contain bacteria, such as salmonella, that cause food poisoning. These foods require special handling in order to prevent the organisms from multiplying to large enough numbers to cause problems. All utensils used in the preparation of meat, including knives and cutting boards, should be cleaned thoroughly with hot soapy water immediately. The organisms are killed during cooking, but vegetables or cooked meat can be infected on a contaminated board or with a dirty knife. If cooked meat is recontaminated in this manner and then made into a sandwich kept all morning in an unrefrigerated lunch bag, the bacteria will have reached very high levels. You and your family do not always have the flu when you think you do. You may have poisoned yourselves.

It is more important for meat-eaters than for vegetarians to observe sanitary habits in the kitchen. It is also necessary to keep meat thoroughly chilled as much of the time as possible. Fresh meat should be cooked before you have had it longer than two days even if you do not plan to use it right away.

Of all meats, liver is the most important to avoid. It is true liver contains all the B vitamins and iron. However, it is extremely high in cholesterol. A 4 ounce serving of liver contains more than 3½ times the maximum amount of cholesterol we should get each day. It also contains many fat-soluble poisons. Cadmium is toxic when large quantities are consumed. It is used in phosphate fertilizers and is taken up by plants, especially cereals. When animals consume these contaminated grains, there is a high concentration of cadmium stored in their livers. All the nutrients available in liver can be obtained from other sources. In addition to liver, other organ meats should be avoided because they are rather high in fat and extremely high in cholesterol content.

Do not eat processed meat like weiners, sausage or bologna. These meats contain huge quantities of fat, plus nitrates, salt, sugar, coloring and many chemicals.

Many people wonder whether it is mandatory to include meat in the diet to maintain optimum health. Vegetarians are not only adequately nourished but their diet puts them at a lower risk of developing many diseases. Vegetarians get much less colon and breast cancer. They have lower blood levels of cholesterol and fats, protecting them against heart disease. They consume less fats and cholesterol, and there are substances such as fiber and phytosterols in plant foods which have cholesterol lowering properties. Animal proteins tend to raise cholesterol levels more than plant proteins.

Beef, pork, and lamb should be used sparingly—more as a condiment than a main dish. Simply cook small pieces of meat along with vegetables or grains. Even lean cuts of meat contain large amounts of fat and cholesterol. Remember that approximately 70 to 80% of the calories from a steak are in the form of fat and only 20 to 30% is from protein.

NUTS AND SEEDS

Nuts and seeds are whole natural foods containing protein and many valuable minerals and vitamins. They should only be eaten in small amounts because they have a high oil content. They were eaten by early man—the "hunter-gatherer." However, man at that time was not sedentary. In addition, nuts and seeds were seasonal so they were eaten infrequently and in small quantities.

If your triglycerides are low, 3 or 4 nuts a day won't hurt you. They should not, of course, be roasted in oil, sugared, or salted. It is best to buy unshelled nuts for two reasons. The nut meats will not be exposed to the air and become rancid and you will not eat as many when you have to shell them yourself. The shells discourage overindulgence.

Small amounts of little seeds—caraway, poppy, celery, and sesame—can be used in baking, salad dressings, or as condiments. They have a tough outer coating and we don't completely chew them. Therefore, we do not absorb much of the fat they contain. Tahini, sesame seeds pulverized into a paste, contains a very large amount of readily available oil accounting for 83% of the calories.

Remember, nuts and seeds are similar to grains in protein but they are high fat foods. About 80% of the total calories of nuts and seeds is from fat, compared to about 5 to 15% for grains. The following charts will allow you to compare the similarity in their protein amounts and the vast differences in their fat contents.

NUTS, SEEDS AND GRAINS
CALORIE, PROTEIN, FAT AND CARBOHYDRATE CONTENT
PER 100 GRAMS (3½ OZ.)

	CALORIES	PROTEIN		FAT		CARBOHYDRATE	
	Calories	Grams	Percent of Calories	Grams	Percent of Calories	Grams	Percent of Calories
NUTS & SEEDS							
ALMONDS	598	18.6	10.8%	54.2	75.9%	19.5	13.3%
BRAZIL NUTS	654	14.3	7.6	66.9	85.6	10.9	6.8
COCONUT, FRESH	346	3.5	3.5	35.3	85.4	9.4	11.1
COCONUT, DRIED UNSWEETENED	662	7.2	3.8	64.9	82.1	23.0	14.1
COCONUT, DRIED SWEENTENED	548	3.6	2.3	39.1	59.7	53.2	38.0
LYCHEES, RAW	64	.9	4.9	0.3	3.9	16.4	91.2
LYCHEES, DRIED	277	3.8	4.8	1.2	3.6	70.7	91.6
MACADAMIA	691	7.8	3.9	71.6	86.7	15.9	9.4
PEANUTS*	582	26.2	15.6	48.7	70.0	20.6	14.4
PUMPKIN SEEDS	553	29.0	18.2	46.7	70.7	15.0	11.1
SESAME SEEDS	582	18.2	10.9	53.4	76.8	17.6	12.3
SUNFLOWER SEEDS	560	24.0	14.9	47.3	70.7	19.9	14.4
WALNUTS, BLACK	628	20.5	11.3	59.3	79.0	14.8	9.7
WALNUTS, ENGLISH	651	14.8	7.9	64.0	82.3	15.8	9.8
WATER CHESTNUTS	79	1.4	6.1	0.2	2.1	19.0	91.8

GRAINS

BARLEY	349	8.2	8.3	1.0	2.4	78.8	89.3
BUCKWHEAT FLOUR,							
DARK	333	11.7	11.8	2.5	6.3	72.0	81.9
OATMEAL, DRY	390	14.2	12.6	7.4	15.9	68.2	71.5
OATMEAL, COOKED	55	2.0	12.6	1.0	15.2	9.7	72.2
RICE, BROWN, RAW	360	7.5	7.1	1.9	4.4	77.4	88.5
RICE, BROWN,							
COOKED	119	2.5	7.2	0.6	4.2	25.5	88.6
RYE, WHOLE GRAIN	334	12.1	11.0	1.7	4.3	73.4	84.7
WHEAT, WHOLE							
GRAIN	330	14.0	15.2	2.2	5.6	69.1	79.2
WHOLE WHEAT							
FLOUR	333	13.3	14.3	2.0	5.0	71.0	80.7

*PEANUTS ARE ACTUALLY LEGUMES AND NOT NUTS, BUT HAVE A FAT CONTENT SIMILAR TO NUTS.

OILS

How should we cut down on our intake of fats? As little extracted oils as possible should be used. Oils, as well as fats, are harmful to the arteries. If they oxidize—become rancid—they cause the destruction of many vitamins. Vitamin E prevents the oxidation of oils, but this vitamin is partially destroyed when oils are refined or hydrogenated. Heated polyunsaturated fats generate peroxides which destroy vitamin E. Extracted oils are heated in processing and are, therefore, potentially more toxic than fresh oils occurring in whole foods. Even if they are "cold-pressed" these oils are run through steel mills and become hot. We should obtain the necessary oils from whole foods. Ample amounts are provided in vegetables, grains, and legumes. Even plant sources can provide excessive amounts of fats in the diet if too much of the wrong kinds are eaten, for instance olives and avocados. Most plant foods contain 1 to 10% fat or less, but avocados contain 88% and should be eaten only rarely.

However, it is better to eat vegetables high in oils than to eat the oils that have been extracted from them. Food prepared by nature is more apt to be balanced than food prepared by a commercial processor. Let me give you an example. Grains, legumes, nuts and seeds contain oils high in unsaturated fatty acids including the essential linoleic acid. They are high also in vitamin E which prevents rancidity. When we extract these oils, we do not get the necessary vitamin E that we would if we ate the whole food. The more vegetable oils we use, the higher our need for vitamin E. We would not have to worry about things like this if we would eat whole foods instead of partitioning them and eating only certain parts.

Margarines are made from vegetable oils. The oils are partially hydrogenated—rendered saturated—to make them solid. This is done using nickel as a catalyst and it is too expensive for the processors to remove the nickel that contaminates their product. Excessive amounts of nickel alter lipid metabolism. It has been shown, in rabbit studies, to cause an increase in plasma lipids. In addition, during the hydrogenation process, some of the fatty acids are converted into forms (trans fatty acids) which do not naturally occur in vegetable oils. These altered fatty acids cause an increase in cholesterol and fats in the blood, contributing to the development of atherosclerosis and cancer. They also tend to cause deficiency of linoleic acid (the essential fatty acid) and have adverse effects on the cells. Less expensive margarines, dairy creamers and toppings are frequently made from palm or coconut oils because they are cheap. These oils are 99% saturated—more saturated than the fat in meat or butterfat. Sometimes even these oils are further hydrogenated in the manufacture of margarine. Many people mistakenly consume these products in an attempt to replace saturated fats in their diets. Avoid using margarine as a spread or in cooking. Sauté vegetables in water instead of oil. In making soups, cut the vegetables up and add them shortly before serving. The result will be a fresher tasting soup.

In general, try to substitute healthier recipes for those you are now using. If you really like a certain food prepared by frying, try baking it instead. Foods should not be fried for three reasons. The first is it increases the fat content of the food. Secondly, it causes foods to be heated to extreme temperatures destroying heat labile nutrients. Thirdly, when oils or fats are heated high enough to smoke, the fat decomposes and irritants suspected of causing cancer are produced. One of these irritants is acrolein which is derived from the glycerol portion of the fat molecule. It is a strong irritant to skin and mucous membranes. When vegetable oils are brought to high temperatures, they join together forming large molecules and can turn to varnish. Now you know what that varnish-like substance is on the bottom of your electric frying pan, wok or popcorn popper.

POULTRY

Poultry is somewhat lower in cholesterol and a good deal lower in fat than other animal foods. The light meat is especially low in fat content. For this reason, it is best to use the breast of chicken or turkey. The skin contains a large amount of fat and should be removed before cooking. When you buy chicken, have the butcher remove the skin and bones. Keep the bones in a plastic bag in the freezer until you have accumulated enough to make stock. I buy from a butcher shop that carries chicken free from hormones and many other undesirable substances.

To make stock, cover the bones with water. Add a little vinegar to help leach the calcium from the bones into the broth. For additional flavor you can add vegetables, bay leaf, and a few peppercorns. Cook slowly all day. In order to save energy, you can cook them for a shorter period in a pressure cooker. When the stock is cool enough to handle, pour it through a colander into a large container. Then fill straight-sided jars with the stock and refrigerate. The fat will rise to the top and solidify. Be sure to remove all of it before using the stock. You can keep stock for a long time in the freezer. If you only use small amounts at a time, pour the stock (after the fat has been removed) into an ice cube tray. When frozen, put the stock cubes into a plastic bag and keep in the freezer. If you have no bones for making stock, you can use chicken wings. This stock can be used in place of all or part of the water when making soups and stews or cooking vegetables.

Steaming is a good way to cook chicken. Inexpensive, collapsible, stainless steel steamers are available. They fit almost any size pot and can be used to steam many foods. Chicken can also be cooked in a microwave oven or it can be wrapped in foil and baked in the oven. The cooked chicken can be eaten just as it is, it can be "creamed" as in the tuna recipe and served on rice or pasta, or it can be added to vegetables or soups.

Chicken Stew on Noodles

1 lb. whole wheat ribbons (noodles made without eggs; whole wheat spaghetti may be substituted)
1 whole chicken breast, raw and cut into small pieces
3-4 carrots, cut into ¾" chunks
1 bay leaf
1½ cups chopped onions, ¾" chunks
4 stalks celery with leaves, ¾" chunks
6-8 cloves garlic, pressed
½ pound mushrooms, sliced (optional)
juice of 1 lemon (approx. ¼ to ⅓ cup)
½ tsp. each marjoram, rosemary (crushed)
¼ tsp. white pepper
heaping ⅓ cup whole wheat flour
2 cups chicken broth

Mix flour and stock in blender. Set aside. Get out spices and measuring spoons. Crush rosemary. Cut chicken. Squeeze lemon. Put large pot of water on to boil for cooking noodles. Cook noodles while continuing. Cook carrots in small sauce pan in 1½ cups water with a bay leaf. Separately cook all the other vegetables in 3 tbs. water in a large, heavy covered skillet for 10 minutes. Add water drained from carrots to flour mixture and blend again. Set aside. Add spices and chicken to skillet. Sauté 2 minutes or just until chicken turns from pink to white. Add flour mixture and carrots, turn up heat and stir until it boils for one minute. Add lemon juice. Spoon a little of chicken stew over cooked ribbons and serve. Combine left-over stew with ribbons so they will not stick together.
Serves 4.

SPICES

Spices are the aromatic parts (fruit, seeds, bark, root or flowers) of plants used to season foods. Herbs are the flavorful leaves of plants used for the same purpose. The flavor and aroma of spices are due to the essential oils they contain. These oils also contain substances which in large amounts could be toxic. Different spices are irritating to varying degrees. Studies have shown they can cause damage to the cells of the gastrointestinal tract with which they come in contact. When yeasts are exposed to the more irritating spices, their growth is inhibited initially, but they quickly adapt. This may also be the case with humans.

The more irritating spices—hot peppers, ginger and black pepper—can cause greater harm and some spices may even be mutagenic. However, they are more apt to do damage in people who are malnourished. Unfortunately, it is in countries where food is scarce that many of these spices are used in large amounts.

The irritating quality of "hot" spices causes them to act as expectorants making your nose run and thinning out mucus so it can be coughed up from the bronchial tubes. Hot chilies and cayenne pepper also increase the flow of blood in superficial blood vessels. These two effects account for the temporary relief from congestion of colds and sinusitis when you eat in a Mexican restaurant.

Many herbs and spices may affect the mind as well. Most people won't ingest or smoke celery seeds, morning glory seeds, paprika or cinnamon sticks. However, they might consume toxic amounts of nutmeg, a psychoactive drug that can cause hallucinations. It also causes unpleasant side effects such as headache, cramps, dry mouth, nausea, tachycardia (rapid beating of the heart), dizziness and constipation. Since the account in Malcolm X's autobiography of the use of nutmeg in jail, the government has eliminated mace and nutmeg in the kitchens of federal penal institutions. Nutmeg is a seed and mace is the network-like covering which encloses it. The taste of the two spices is similar.

People seek out plants for their psychogenic properties and animals do, too. Cats, for instance, enjoy smelling, eating and rolling in catnip, sometimes called catmint. It is a member of the mint (Labateae) family along with peppermint, spearmint, sage, marjoram, thyme and pennyroyal. The flavor and aroma of these plants are due to essential oils secreted by glands which can be seen under a microscope lens as translucent dots on the leaves. Unlike the other members of the mint family, catnip contains a substance possessing mild narcotic properties which is what attracts cats.

Spices make the art of cooking more enjoyable. Seasonings make it easier to prepare tasty meals without using harmful fats, sweeteners or salt. Spices are used in only very small quantities; we use even smaller amounts of the more irritating ones because they taste hotter or stronger. Adequate fiber in the diet protects the mucous membranes of the gastrointestinal tract against the irritating effects of many substances including spices. The best policy is to use moderation when it comes to spices.

SPICES

Irritating	Mild	Non-Irritating
Cayenne Pepper	Allspice[3]	Caraway Seeds
Cloves	Anise	Celery Seeds
Ginger[1]	Cinnamon	Dill Seeds[4]
Horseradish	Coriander	Fennel Seeds
Mustard Seed	Cumin	Paprika
Pepper (Black and white)[2]	Mace	Saffron[5]
	Nutmeg	Turmeric

[1] Ginger is a rhizome, an underground stem that sends shoots above ground.

[2] Peppercorns are white at first and turn red when ripe. Black pepper is made from the sun-dried peppercorns, the skin of which turns black when dried. White pepper, which has a milder taste, is made from peppercorns from which the skin has first been removed.

[3] Contrary to common belief, allspice is not a combination of spices. It comes from the berry of a tree of the myrtle family.

[4] Dill is a member of the carrot family. The seeds are used as a spice and the leaves as an herb in flavoring foods.

[5] Saffron is the dried stigmas of the purple flower of the crocus. It is used both to flavor and color foods and formerly was used as a dye. Since the stigma is very tiny and must be collected by hand, saffron is quite expensive.

Herbs come from the leaves of plants. They tend to be sweet and non-irritating. They include:

Herbs

Basil	Oregano
Bay leaf	Rosemary
Dill Weed	Sage
Fennel	Savory
Marjoram	Tarragon
Mint (Peppermint and Spearmint)	Thyme

Chili powder is not a single spice but a blend of ground chili peppers, cumin, oregano, garlic, black pepper, coriander, salt and sometimes allspice and cloves. Pure ground chili peppers for use in Mexican cooking can be found in some supermarkets; it is not called chili powder but *mulato* or *pasilla*.

Curry is also a combination of spices. In India, there is a wide variety of curries. In our country, curry is made of cinnamon, coriander, ginger, mace, nutmeg, pepper and mainly turmeric, which gives it the characteristic color.

SUGAR

Table sugar is a highly concentrated and unnatural food. It takes huge quantities of sugar cane or beets to make a very small amount of sucrose. Most natural foods contain adequate amounts of the nutrients necessary for their metabolism. In refining sugar beets and cane, 90% of the plant is removed along with the vitamins and minerals needed to help the body utilize the sugar. These nutrients activate enzyme systems that break down food. Although these nutrients occur only in small amounts, their absence forces the body to draw on its reserves in order to assimilate the nutrient-depleted foods. This can lead to deficiencies. Dr. Henry Schroeder, an expert in the study of minerals, says that white sugar is devoid of all the trace elements necessary for its metabolism. Of course, sugar from all sources should be taken in extreme moderation. Dark brown sugar is refined sugar with molasses added. It is slightly better than refined sugar since molasses contains the nutrients that have been removed from the sugar. It is, however, a concentrated food completely lacking in bulk and is much too rapidly assimilated. Raw sugar cannot be sold in the United States since it contains many impurities including soil, molds and insect parts. Turbinado sugar is not as completely refined as white sugar so it is not quite as bad—but almost.

Natural sources of sugar are undesirable but less so than processed sugar. These natural forms include pure maple syrup, sorghum and honey. Honey contains the nutrients necessary for its metabolism. It is natural in the sense that it is unprocessed by man if the uncooked, unfiltered variety is used. Since it is more than twice as sweet as table sugar you can use less to obtain the same degree of sweetness. However, it has been partially broken down by bees into single sugars and enters the bloodstream quite rapidly. It contains fructose, slightly less glucose, and only a little sucrose (See *Carbohydrates*.) Fructose tastes sweeter than other sugars and this is the reason for the sweetness of honey.

Honey shouldn't be given to babies under one year of age. About 10% of honey contains spores of the bacteria, *Clostridium botulinum*, which produce a virulent toxin causing botulism. In adults the spores are harmless. The intestinal climate of some infants, however, is such that when the spores are ingested, the toxin can be formed in the body. Most of the cases of infant botulism seen in this country in recent years have been traced to honey containing botulism spores. Many of the afflicted babies died. Under no circumstances should honey be given to babies since the spores are not destroyed by cooking.

Pure maple syrup is another natural sugar, and therefore, better than table sugar. But like honey and molasses, it should be used only in lieu of white sugar when you are determined to use a sweetener of some kind.

Molasses is not a natural product, but is a result of refining sugar cane or beets. It contains all the nutrients that were extracted in a concentrated form, although not terribly many were there originally. I like to use a little, though, when I make bread because the yeast will feed on the sugar and leave the nutrients for me.

SUGAR CONTENT OF SOME COMMONLY USED PROCESSED FOODS

Food	Percent of Sugar
Jello	82.6
Coffee-Mate	65.4
Cremora	56.9
Hershey Milk Chocolate	51.4
Shake 'n Bake (Barbeque Style)	50.9
Sara Lee Chocolate Cake	35.9
Wish Bone Russian Dressing	30.2
Heinz Tomato Catsup	28.9
Quaker 100% Natural Cereal	23.9
Wish Bone Sweet 'n Spicy French Dressing	23.0
Hamburger Helper	23.0
Sealtest Chocolate Ice Cream	21.4
Cool Whip	21.0
Libby's Canned Peach Halves	17.9
Shake 'n Bake (Original Flavor)	17.4
Wyler's Beef Flavor Bouillon Cubes	14.8
Shake 'n Bake (Italian Style)	14.7
Dannon Lowfat Blueberry Yogurt	13.7
Ritz Crackers	11.8
Del Monte Canned Corn	10.7
Skippy Creamy Peanut Butter	9.2
Coca-Cola	8.8*
Wish Bone Italian Salad Dressing	7.3
Ragu Spaghetti Sauce	6.2

* This figure may seem low because most of Coke is water. If we figure the amount of sugar on the basis of percent of total calories rather than percent by weight, Coke would be about 100% sugar.

Of the many forms of carbohydrate available in the supermarket, refined white sugar is the worst form one can choose. However, all simple carbohydrates are harmful if eaten in more than limited amounts. Candy bars or bakery products purchased in a health food store are just as harmful as these same products purchased in an ordinary market.

In addition to the sugar we add to foods in the home, we consume a great amount of hidden sugar. Actually, most of the sugar we eat is in processed foods. Twenty-four percent of our calories come from sugar; 3% come from fruits and vegetabls and 3% from milk sugar (lactose). The rest is hidden in processed foods. We often are not aware of the amount of sugar added to many commonly used foods. I have listed some of these foods and the percentage of sugar they contain in the chart above.

Sugar is even added to dog food. It is also added to baby foods and ready-to-eat breakfast cereals. Some brands of cereal list the different kinds of sugar separately on the label. Sucrose might be the third ingredient with other kinds of sugar appearing toward the end of the list. If they were all lumped together as total sugar, it would often have to be listed as the first ingredient, followed by wheat, corn or rice.

Although the amount of sucrose consumed annually in the United States has remained about the same for the past fifty years, the amount of other sugars—mainly corn syrup used in the food industry—has been increasing. From 1960 to 1977 our consumption of sugar derived from corn starches climbed from 13 to 32 pounds per person per year. Sugar is replacing complex carbohydrates in the diet. As the amount of sugar we eat rises higher and higher, the amount of starches continues to decline.

If you want a sweetener in your cooking, try using whole natural foods. Many foods are naturally quite sweet: carrots, beets, sweet potatoes and almost all fruits. Learn to make use of these foods to obtain the sweetness.

The artificial sweetener, saccharine, has been found to cause cancer of the bladder in laboratory animals. A report showed the risk of bladder cancer in men and in women using tabletop artificial sweetener (that not in prepared foods) was higher than for those who do not use it. Although saccharine itself is only a weak carcinogen, it may be a cancer "promoter." That means it increases the chances that a carcinogen will cause cancer. We do not know much about the additives or contaminants in prepared foods. It is prudent to avoid this substance that could enhance our chance of developing cancer.

A new artificial sweetener, Aspartame, made from amino acids is about 200 times sweeter than sugar. It is presently being tested. If approved, it will be an ingredient in dry beverage mixes and will also be available as a tabletop sweetener but will not be used in diet sodas.

VEGETABLES

Vegetables are the edible flowers, stems, leaves and roots of plants. They have a high water content and are, therefore, low in calories. In spite of this, they contain generous amounts of a wide variety of nutrients. In addition they provide a valuable source of fiber. Although vegetables contain many of the same nutrients found in grains and legumes, it is essential they be included in the diet as they are rich in vitamins C and A. Unlike fruit, vegetables contain only small amounts of sugar so they can be eaten in unlimited quantities. Care should be taken to eat deep yellow, orange and green colored vegetables several times a week because they supply the precursor from which vitamin A is made in the body. Vitamin A is a vitamin missing in grains, although it is found in legumes in modest amounts.

Some raw or lightly cooked vegetables should be eaten every day. Steaming is a good way to cook them. If they are boiled in water, the resulting broth should be used in soups, stews or other foods.

Fresh vegetables are best if good quality produce is available. Such is not the case in all seasons, in all parts of the country. Vegetables fresh from the garden or farm are preferable to vegetables from the supermarket. The leafy vegetables loose much of their vitamin content when stored, particularly if they are allowed to wilt. Excessive spraying with water in the market will cause a loss of water soluble vitamins.

Frozen vegetables are picked at the height of ripeness when the vitamin content is highest, and they are often flash frozen in the fields. At times, frozen vegetables contain more vitamins than fresh ones. If, however, they are not maintained at optimum temperatures during shipping, loading and storage they will lose nutrients. Canned vegetables should be used as seldom as possible. They have been heated and contain added salt and sugar and usually other additives as well.

Stir "Fry" Vegetables

Cooked brown rice
About 2 cups cut up vegetables
Your choice of several of the following or any others (more if using cabbage or sprouts as they cook down):

1 onion, halved and sliced
2 stalks celery, thinly sliced on the diagonal
1 small or ½ large head cauliflower broken into flowerettes
1 stalk broccoli, cut off top into flowerettes, slice branched part of stalk, peel remainder of stalk and cut into long slender pieces
1-2 carrots, sliced on diagonal, stacked and cut into matchsticks

Brussels sprouts cut into halves, then cut each half into quarters
⅛-¼ lb. sliced mushrooms or 1 or 2 dried Japanese mushrooms
Raw sweet potato cut into long slender pieces
½ head cabbage, shredded or use Chinese cabbage or bok choy
Green or red bell pepper, sliced
Zucchini
Bean sprouts
¼ lb. snow peas
Frozen peas

Sauce:
3 tbs. soy sauce
2 tbs. corn starch
¼ cup water
2-3 paper thin slices fresh ginger (optional)
⅛-¼ tsp. black pepper or crushed dry chili peppers (optional)

Mix the sauce ingredients in a small bowl. Fold ginger slices in quarters and put through garlic press into sauce. Set aside. Prepare the vegetables for cooking. In a large heavy pot heat ¼ cup water over moderately high heat, add onions and Brussels sprouts and steam, covered, 1 minute. Add other vegetables except sprouts or snow peas. Stir, using 2 large wooden spoons. Cover and steam 3 minutes. Add sprouts, stir and steam 1 minute. Add snow peas. Stir. Remove from heat, stir sauce and add. Mix thoroughly and again place pot on heat, stirring rapidly until thickened. Serve over hot rice.

One of the best ways to serve vegetables, of course, is in a salad. The main problem with salads is the dressing; it usually contains fats and oils. Therefore, I am including examples of two salads that are made with acceptable dressings.

String Bean Salad

1 lb. cooked string beans, fresh or frozen (do not overcook)
⅛ head red cabbage, shredded
Few radishes, sliced
1 carrot. Slice on the diagonal. Then stack slices and cut into matchsticks.

Combine the vegetables. Add ½ cup dressing and toss.

Dressing:

> 2 cups nonfat yogurt
> Juice of ½ lemon or lime
> 3 cloves garlic, pressed
> 2–3 green onions, minced

Stir the ingredients together.

Cucumber and Radish Salad

1 cucumber, peeled and sliced
3–4 radishes, sliced

1-2 tbs. parsley, minced
⅛ tsp. dry mustard
½ tsp. soy sauce
1 pinch black pepper
2 tbs. vinegar

Mix mustard and soy sauce. Add vinegar and pepper. Pour over salad and toss. Steamed broccoli is also good tossed with a little of this sauce.

It is sometimes convenient to use prepared salad dressings. There are some on the market without oil, although they tend to be salty and contain artificial sweeteners. They can be diluted with water, lemon juice and/or vinegar.

Carrots: Vegetables are fairly good sources of fiber although they do not contain as much as grains or legumes. Some vegetables contain more than others including peas, cabbage, winter squash, and carrots. Carrots are one of the best foods to eat if you are afflicted with constipation. Eighty to 90% of their dry weight is fiber and it holds up to five times its weight in water.

Carrots are wonderful vegetables. Because they contain a generous amount of natural sugar, most people like them. They are inexpensive, store well and are available all year. Although they contain many vitamins and are an excellent source of calcium and other minerals, the most valuable nutrient they contain is carotene, the precursor from which vitamin A is formed. People who eat highly processed and fast foods do not usually get enough of this vitamin. For this reason, it is a good idea to keep carrots on hand. Some people prepare carrot sticks and keep them in water in the refrigerator so they are crisp and ready to eat at all times. Don't worry about this causing a loss of nutrients; this method of storing carrots may actually result in less vitamin loss as it prevents the carrots from drying out which will cause oxidation of vitamin A.

Although cooking can destroy some of the nutrients in vegetables, cooking, pureeing or mashing carrots breaks the cell walls making carotene more available for absorption.

Garlic: There does not seem to be a middle of the road when it comes to garlic. People either like it or have an aversion to it. If you are one of those who like it, you are lucky as there are substances in this potent-smelling bulb that have many beneficial effects. Modern scientists haven't proved that it affords protection against vampires, but they have shown that it lowers the amount of cholesterol, triglycerides and sugar in the blood and it decreases the tendency of the blood to form clots. These effects serve to protect against atherosclerosis. Like some of the spices, it works as an expectorant, combatting nasal and bronchial congestion. It also contains sulfur-containing substances that have antibiotic properties against many kinds of bacteria. Some preliminary and inconclusive research indicates that garlic may increase the immunity of mice to cancer.

The benefits of garlic are so diverse that it is now available in health food stores. However, if you don't like garlic, don't eat it. If you like it, invest in a good garlic press. A good press is effective and will eliminate the necessity of peeling the garlic. This will not only save time, but prevent those garlic fingers. (If you do get garlic on your hands, wet them and rub them with salt before washing with soap and water.) Some presses are even self-cleaning. Buy loose garlic because it tends to be fresher than the kind found in packages. When sautéing garlic and onions, use a little water instead of oil or butter. Besides avoiding fat, you will be less apt to brown the garlic. To insure fresh breath after enjoying garlic, chew a sprig of parsley or a clove bud.

Lettuce: Most leafy vegetables contain almost every known nutrient and are low in calories and fat. Lettuce is an excellent food, is available year-round, and has a milder taste than many leafy vegetables. Because it is eaten raw, nutrients are not lost in the cooking water. In addition, it does not have the high oxalate content of many other greens so that the calcium it contains is readily absorbed.

Most people buy Iceberg lettuce but Romaine is better as it contains more of most nutrients. Below is a chart showing the nutritional value of these two types of lettuce.

NUTRITION VALUE OF ROMAINE & ICEBURG LETTUCE—PER 100 GRAMS

	Water	Calories	Protein	Fat	Carbohydrates	Fiber	Ash	Tryptophan	Lysine	Methionine
Romaine Lettuce	94%	18	1.3g	.3g	3.5g	.7g	.9g	13mg	75mg	4mg
Iceberg Lettuce	95.5%	13	.9g	.1g	2.9g	.5g	.6g	12mg	70mg	4mg

	Calcium	Phosph.	Iron	Sodium	Potassium	Vitamin A.	Thiamine	Ribo.	Niacin	Vitamin C
Romaine Lettuce	68mg	25mg	1.4mg	9mg	264mg	1900IU	.05mg	.08mg	.4mg	18mg
Iceberg Lettuce	20mg	22mg	.5mg	9mg	175mg	330IU	.06mg	.06mg	.3mg	6mg

Onions: Like garlic, onions contain essential oils rich in sulfur-containing compounds. The disulfides are volatile and are responsible for the characteristic odor. The thiosulfates have antibiotic properties. Factors in the oil of onions offer a degree of protection against fat-induced increases in blood cholesterol and decrease the tendency of the blood to clot, thereby deterring the formation of arterial plaques. The same substances that are found in garlic occur in lesser concentrations in onions. If you are eating fats or fatty foods, eating onions or garlic may minimize their undesirable effects.

Potatoes: The common potato is a fairly good source of protein, vitamins and minerals. It is a very good source of vitamin C but the content of this vitamin decreases during storage. Potatoes are low in fat and are not fattening. It is the high-fat toppings that add calories.

The potato is a member of the nightshade family (Solanaceae) along with the deadly nightshade plant. Members of this family contain alkaloid toxins, especially solanine, which is found in all parts of the plant. It is usually quite low in the tuber or potato itself but is concentrated in the eyes. For this reason, care should be taken to remove the eyes before cooking.

Sometimes potatoes have a greenish coloring because they have grown too close to the surface of the soil. This causes a high concentration of solanine in the skin due to the action of sunlight. These potatoes should be discarded or the green areas carefully pared away. Greening of potatoes can occur during prolonged storage in supermarkets due to the action of the fluorescent lighting. For this reason, potatoes are often packaged in brown plastic bags, but this measure is not always effective. Potatoes should be stored in a dry, dark place. Those that have sprouted should be discarded.

Large amounts of potatoes should not be purchased unless they are to be used within a reasonable period of time. If exposed to light during storage or if stored for prolonged periods, solanine accumulation may reach levels toxic to man.

In the fall of 1969, 78 British schoolboys were poisoned after eating potatoes left over from the summer term. Diarrhea, vomiting and abdominal pain were experienced seven to 19 hours after the meal. Other symptoms were trembling, muscle spasm, convulsive twitching, calf pain, dizziness, blurred vision, dehydration, difficulty in breathing, hallucinations, stupor and coma. The potatoes eaten by the boys had been peeled, but when the solanine content is high enough, it diffuses throughout the tuber.

There have been many incidents of the poisoning of both humans and livestock by unfit potatoes. The problem was expecially severe in Korea between 1952 and 1953 when many people died after subsisting on rotten potatoes.

Wounds or injuries elicit a response in potatoes that causes the formation of the alkaloids so that only unblemished potatoes should be purchased. For this reason, potatoes should not be peeled or cut until ready to be cooked. They especially should not be peeled and left in the light.

Fortunately, the government monitors the amount of solanine in potatoes, and species that produce higher amounts have been removed from the market. Although this reduces the danger of poisoning, it does not eliminate the necessity of taking precautions.

Squash: Squashes, pumpkins and cucumbers are really fruits, and like melons thay all belong to the gourd family. Squash is native to America. The hard-shelled winter varieties were especially important to the Indians since they could be stored for relatively long periods of time. Squash is a good source of carotene.

A good way to prepare acorn or other kinds of hard-shelled squash is to cut them in half and remove the seeds. Turn cut side down and steam until just barely tender. Scoop out the pulp and mash with a diced apple, a squeeze of lemon juice and a little cinnamon. Return pulp to shells and bake for 15 to 20 minutes at 350°.

Sweet Potatoes: There are many varieties of sweet potatoes, varying in color. They can be very pale, a deep orange or purple. They contain a great deal of vitamin A, the darker varieties containing more than the lighter ones. The darker sweet potatoes are quite often mistakenly called yams. They are moister when cooked than the lighter ones and quite a bit sweeter.

Mechanical injury and molds can cause the formation of toxins. Moldy sweet potatoes have been the cause of substantial loss of livestock. Only firm, unblemished potatoes should be purchased. If you find, after cooking, that a potato has rotten areas, they should be carefully cut away. The unblemished part will be uncontaminated.

Sweet potatoes are sweet and moist when baked. They are a colorful and delicious addition to vegetables. They are also very good when thinly sliced and eaten raw.

Yams: Yams are grown mostly in the tropics and are not found in markets in the United States, although they do grow to a limited extent in Louisiana and Florida. The darker colored varieties of the sweet potato are frequently and erroneously called yams in this country, but they belong to a different family.

Yeast: Yeasts are microscopic plants. Brewer's yeast converts carbohydrates to alcohol; baker's yeast converts carbohydrates to carbon dioxide, a gas which causes bread to rise. Yeasts can be dried and used as a flavoring agent in prepared foods or as a protein and vitamin supplement.

Brewer's yeast and Torula yeast are usually used as supplements. Yeasts do not normally contain vitamin B_{12}, but they can assimilate it from the

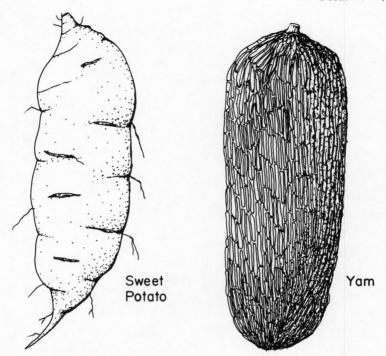

Sweet
Potato

Yam

culture on which they are grown. If necessary, additional nutrients are added before packaging to meet label standards.

Yeasts contain large amounts of substances that are converted to uric acid in the body. In some people, consuming foods high in these substances results in an undesirably high level of uric acid in the blood.

Torula yeast is sometimes grown on hydrocarbon petroleum products instead of carbohydrates. Since many hydrocarbons are carcinogenic, Japan, Great Britain and Italy have withheld approval of this yeast. The United States has been producing 15 million pounds of this kind of yeast a year since 1975. It is used in bakery and meat products, frozen foods and baby foods. It is used in large quantities in foods served in restaurants, hotels and schools.

Yeast is high in protein: 50 to 60% of its calories are in protein. This is too high for a healthful diet, unless consumed in small amounts.

I hope the recipes and information in this chapter are helpful in showing you how food can be prepared with a greatly reduced intake of fats, sugars and salt. The technique of preparing recipes is more important than the ingredients. You should not become overly dependent on other people's recipes but learn to create your own. Once you have tried these recipes, I think you will find it easier to start experimenting on your own. You can also adapt favorites you already use. Be on the watch for new recipes that lend themselves to conversion to this way of cooking.

Chapter 3

HOW TO LOSE WEIGHT

When losing weight, the kind of food you eat is more important than how much you eat. Learn which foods are high in bulk and low in calories. Creative food preparation can make these foods appealing. For many people, losing weight is the hardest thing they've ever done. I will discuss many aspects of this problem. People can control their weight and eat a more healthful diet at the same time.

CHANGE YOUR METABOLISM

You will be able to lose a certain amount of weight simply by eating a healthful diet. However, exercise is also an important aspect of a weight loss program. Americans are getting fatter because they have become more sedentary. Besides "burning off" more calories, exercise will cause a change in your metabolism. It will cause a shift in the proportion of your food that is converted to energy rather than to fat. To convert food, as well as the fat stored in our bodies, to energy we need a good deal of oxygen. Exercising increases the amount of oxygen taken to the cells so this can take place. That is why we feel more energetic after exercising. Many fat people are lethargic because thay cannot produce enough energy.

Exercise also causes the secretion of epinephrine (adrenaline) which acts as an appetite suppressant. Although short periods of light exercise can make you hungry, a half hour or more of brisk exercise has the opposite effect. Twenty-five years ago, nutritionist Jean Mayer showed that food intake decreases with a certain level of physical activity. By the same token, activity below a certain level actually causes an increase in appetite. Inactivity is believed to play an important role in the increased weight of people living in industrialized societies.

Overweight people should walk every day. Walking is more strenuous for people who are carrying a lot of weight than it is for thin people. Don't think of jogging if you are too heavy. Be patient. You will be in better condition sooner than you think. Brisk walking is a fine exercise. Try to do it before your largest meal of the day. This will work as a natural appetite suppressant. Don't overdress when you exercise. The cooler you are when exercising, the more weight you will lose.

If you really want to lose weight, start exercising. At first, the amount of time spent is less important than the fact that you exercise regularly. Exercise will make you feel better about your body and improve your self-esteem even while you are overweight. (See *Exercise*)

HOW MANY CALORIES DO YOU NEED?

While many people in America don't receive adequate nutrients because of poor food choices, it would be difficult to find many who are not getting enough calories. Most people realize they should cut down on their calories, and some want to know how many they should consume. Only you can determine how much food you should eat. You must take personal responsibility for understanding your body. The amount of fuel you need depends on the amount your body burns and this is dependent on many factors.

Body Size and Type: Large bodies require more energy for their operation, but overweight people need less per pound than thinner ones. This is because there is a great deal of metabolic activity taking place in muscle cells. The requirements of fat tissue for oxygen and energy is much lower because the cells of this tissue are a lot less active.

Sex: Women have more body fat in proportion to muscle than men and, therefore, they utilize less energy. For this reason, the resting metabolic rate of women is approximately 5% lower than men's.

Emotional Health: Depression results in a lower expenditure of energy. Tension, on the other hand, causes a greater energy expenditure. Eating is the way some people deal with stress, but the extra energy expended doesn't usually compensate for the additional calories consumed.

Physical Health: During sickness, you burn more calories, especially if you have a fever. The need for calories and for many nutrients is altered when you are sick. For this reason, a special diet may be prescribed during and after a prolonged illness.

Age: The older we are, the fewer calories we require. Older people usually expend fewer calories and lack of exercise causes an increase in fat and a decrease in muscle tissue. Since muscle tissue is more active metabolically, it requires more energy even at rest. Children need more calories per unit of body weight than adults because it requires energy to grow. The basal (resting) metabolic rate increases up to the age of two, then it declines gradually until puberty when it rises again. After puberty it resumes its decline.

Temperature: Because energy is required to maintain a constant internal body temperature, we expend more energy during periods of extreme temperatures, both hot and cold.

Exercise: The more sedentary a person is, the fewer calories are needed. An inactive person may use 1500 calories a day. A very active person may burn 5000 to 7000.

Basal Metabolic Rate: Some people's bodies run at a faster rate and they require more calories at rest than do people whose metabolic rate is lower.

Caloric needs vary widely, not only from person to person, but for the same person under different circumstances. No authority and no height/weight chart can tell you how much and what kind of food you need to eat. You know when you are at your best. You know how you react when you see yourself in the mirror. The most important thing you can learn from this book is to observe yourself, understand, and then take responsibility for yourself.

WHAT TO EAT AND WHEN TO EAT IT

It is especially important for the dieter to eat a large breakfast, one or two morning snacks, a good lunch and an afternoon snack or two. If you don't eat enough your blood sugar will drop and you will feel hungry and tire easily. Cooked cereal is the best choice for breakfast. You can use skim milk on it but don't drink large quantities of milk since it is a fiberless food that contains a lot of sugar (lactose). Lactose isn't as sweet as other sugars, but it contains as many calories as any sugar. Eat a piece of fruit for breakfast but avoid juices. The juices won't fill you up and they will be absorbed too fast causing an increase in insulin. The insulin will cause more fats to be made by the body.

For lunch you can eat banana sandwiches on whole grain bread or crackers, vegetable sandwiches, or left-overs. Avoid dried fruit; it should be fresh. Avoid olives as they contain too much oil, or pickles as they are too salty. Munch *plenty* of cut-up vegetables. To prevent boredom, avoid getting into the celery-and-carrot-stick rut. Try hunks of raw red cabbage, kohlrabi slices, peeled broccoli stems, and water chestnuts. Be imaginative and spend time trying new foods and new ways of preparing them.

In the evening eat a large meal, low in density. Food eaten in the evening must contain a lot of fiber and water. A huge salad is the best choice. Eat it first, it tastes better when you are hungry and you will eat more. You can't eat salad as fast as you can softer foods because it requires so much chewing. It takes about 20 minutes after you start eating, before you begin to feel satisfied. If you eat too fast you will eat more than the amount that would have sufficed if you had eaten slowly.

If you enjoy snacking in the evenings, do so. Buy a hot air popper so you can make popcorn without oil. Popcorn is not especially nutritious but it is a good source of fiber, tastes good, is low in calories, takes a long time to eat and is filling. It is an ideal food for compulsive eaters. Take some in your lunch; serve it to company. Avoid snacking too heavily on fruit since it is high in sugar. When you do eat fruit, make sure it is not too ripe. For instance buy bananas when they are still slightly green, before most of the starch they contain has been converted to sugar. If you eat too much fruit at one time, it will cause an initial rise in your blood sugar and a subsequent drop causing pangs. Several pieces of fruit, however, are better than a handful of peanuts or candy.

Don't let yourself get bored with the food you are eating. Fresh fruit and vegetables have to be bought often. However, canned and frozen foods are full of chemical preservatives, salt, and sugar. Shop often so you always have a *variety* of fresh produce on hand.

Red meat, even the lean cuts, and poultry and fish contain hidden fat. Either eliminate them from your diet, or eat them infrequently. Save them for a special occasion, or when you have company. In general, offer your guests the same food you usually eat. Serving foods that cause disease should not be associated with hospitality. Remember poultry contains less fat than red meat, and the light meat of poultry is leaner than the dark. Steaming is a good way to prepare chicken or fish as it preserves the moistness. You can also bake them in foil, or cook them in the microwave oven.

Don't have fattening foods in the house, they are not good for anyone. Fat people tend to have fat spouses, fat children (natural or adopted) and fat pets.

In addition to the food you eat, supplement the diets of your family with baked potatoes, bread or extra beans, noodles, or rice. If they eat exactly as you do they may lose too much weight. Be sure the extra food they eat is the right kind. Fatty, sweet, refined and highly processed foods are not good for anyone, no matter how much they weigh.

Caffeine: Avoid caffeine. It is a stimulant that causes the secretion of adrenaline. You will experience a temporary elevation of blood sugar after drinking coffee or other caffeine-containing beverages. However, this will be followed by a subsequent drop in blood sugar which will make you feel very hungry. When dieting, *always* avoid hunger.

Gum Chewing: Dieters are often gum chewers but this is a mistake. The chewing action causes the secretion of digestive juices and results in hunger. Keep small pieces of fruit and vegetables handy at all times to satisfy your urge to chew.

Sugar and Spice: Do not use sugar or salt in food preparation, and avoid processed foods that contain them. While your taste buds are adjusting to your diet, the food may seem bland. However, this will keep you from overeating. One reason you became overweight is the seductive way your food has been prepared. It is better to feel full because you have eaten enough plain food, than to feel thwarted because you can eat only a fraction of a dish that is fit for a king. Kings were fat, had gout, and a host of other problems.

Salt causes your body to retain large amounts of water. It will also put you at a greater risk of developing hypertension. If you are overweight, you already risk this dangerous disease. If you think you eat too much salt, never self-medicate with diuretics. They can cause kidney damage. Dramatic diuretic effects can be obtained simply by curtailing salt.

In place of sugar and salt in your meals, make use of herbs and spices. Try to avoid those that irritate the delicate lining of the gastrointestinal tract—mustard, cayenne, pepper, etc.—as they will make you hungrier. Judicious use of spices can make a bland diet more acceptable to the dieter.

Dilute Your Calories: When trying to lose weight you should include as much fiber as possible in your diet. Fiber dilutes digestible, calorie-yielding food; it absorbs water in the stomach and intestines giving you a feeling of fullness; and it takes longer to chew so you feel satisfied before you have eaten too much. Eat whole grains. A slice of whole wheat bread contains slightly less calories than a slice of white bread. However, the whole wheat has four times as much dietary fiber. Limit dairy products because even defatted ones contain no fiber.

HOW FAST SHOULD YOU LOSE WEIGHT?

Don't try to lose weight too rapidly. Dropping pounds quickly can result in an excessive loss of body protein, dehydration, acidosis, and a decrease in glucose tolerance. It can also cause hair loss. Doctors familiar with this phenomenon in people on crash diets say the only treatment is "tincture of time."

It is most important to change the way you are eating. Remember the diet which makes you heavy also causes many diseases. If you learn to enjoy foods that are good for you, you will lose weight slowly and steadily. If you hit a plateau and you haven't been cheating, you will need to re-examine your diet. Either you are eating too much fat or you need to substitute more vegetables for some of the starchier food. The Agriculture Department publishes a book giving the nutrient content of almost all foods. *Nutritive Value of Foods* can be obtained from:

Superintendent of Documents
U.S. Government Printing Office
Washington, D.C.   20402

Send $1.25 and ask for *Home and Garden Bulletin* No. 72. A more comprehensive book, *Nutritive Value of American Foods in Common Units—Agriculture Handbook* No. 456 can be obtained from the same address.

POPULAR WEIGHT REDUCTION REGIMES

Many popular diets have aspects that are definitely unhealthful and actually make it hard for you to lose weight.

High protein/low carbohydrate diets recommend eating large amounts of foods, such as meat, that are high in fat. These diets lack carbohydrate and cause fatigue, irritability, and nausea. The large amount of fat in these diets can also precipitate gouty arthritis, diabetes and hypertension in susceptible people.

Because these diets are low in fiber and high in fat, they will increase your risk of developing diseases of the bowel and many kinds of cancer. Women with benign breast disease would be especially advised to avoid high protein/low carbohydrate diets. They should be avoided by pregnant women who should not lose weight by any method except under the strict supervision of a physician.

Fats cannot be completely metabolized when we do not get enough carbohydrate, consequently these diets cause ketosis. Ketosis is the accumulation of toxic acid substances, ketones. It causes loss of mineral from the bones thereby softening them, a serious problem for overweight people whose skeletons must bear excess weight. Large amounts of water are excreted to remove the ketones from the body, and this can cause dehydration. The initial weight loss on a high protein/low carbohydrate diet is due to dehydration. However, water is necessary for good health and will be regained as soon as you stop dieting.

High protein/low carbohydrate diets also contain large amounts of cholesterol and can lead to the accumulation of plaques in the arteries.

Fats contain more than twice as many calories as carbohydrates. The weight loss on these diets is due to dehydration and cannot be maintained. These diets are expensive, monotonous, ineffective and dangerous. They have been criticized by the medical profession and nutritionists repeatedly and vehemently.

Diets that restrict the amount of food you eat are criticized because of their emotional and physical effects. It isn't pleasant to go through life constantly suppressing one's desire to eat and feeling guilty for those things you do eat. Eating should be wholesome *and* satisfying. Counting calories is difficult and often inaccurate. If you eat the right kinds of food you should have no reason to count calories.

The three-square-meals-a-day-no-snacking diets ignore the fact that eating a few large meals causes the stomach to empty faster resulting in elevated levels of blood sugar followed by low blood sugar and hunger. A fairly constant blood sugar level prevents excessive hunger pangs which can drive you to gorging. Some people even wake up hungry after eating a large, rich dinner. Nibbling causes an increase in glucose tolerance which is an increase in the ability to metabolize carbohydrates. Eating frequently will maintain more normal blood sugar and insulin levels and prevent the sluggish feeling that follows large meals. Eating before you are very hungry will satisfy you with less food and reduce the urge for rich and fattening food.

Frequent eating tends to lower the blood lipids and it has also been observed to improve the overall performance of athletes.

Overeating is an unhealthy extreme, but so is fasting. Fasting results in a greater loss of body protein than of body fat; one-third of a pound of muscle is lost each day during fasting. The fat liberated from the tissues causes the same adverse effects as those of the high protein/low carbohydrate diet.

Some people believe that fasting is a way of cleansing the body of toxins. Actually the kidneys are inhibited in their elimination of toxins during fasting. A much more natural way of detoxifying the body is to eliminate the overconsumption of foods, especially excessive amounts of fats and proteins. Overconsumption of these foods results in the formation and accumulation of metabolites that can be toxic. Another way to assure a "clean" body is to include ample fruit in the diet. Apples and citrus are a rich source of pectins which inhibit the absorption of toxic substances. Pectin also aids in ridding the body of cholesterol.

Prolonged fasting can cause kidney damage, abnormal behavior, brain and nerve damage. Fasting is sometimes used in the case of extreme obesity or in the treatment of allergy. However, studies show it is usually followed by an increase in the weight of obese subjects to higher than prefasting levels. Because it can be dangerous, fasting should only take place under the supervision of a physician.

UNDERSTANDING YOURSELF

In taking care of nutritional needs it is important to get in touch with your own body. Some people feel the need to nibble all day; some are happier eating three meals a day. It isn't wise for a person to force himself to eat when he doesn't want to, or to starve himself when he is hungry. People vary greatly in the size of their stomachs; in the time it takes them to digest; in the quality and amount of digestive enzymes; in the degree to which stress affects their digestion. No set rules would apply to everyone.

You should eat until you feel satisfied and you should eat whenever you have the desire. If you know you can eat when you want to, you will be less likely to feel the compulsion to eat too much at any given time.

The key to weight control is eating the right foods. As you learn what to eat and what not to eat, your tastes will adapt and you will find yourself enjoying things that never interested you before.

Chapter 4

CARBOHYDRATES

Carbohydrates are our main source of fuel. Without the glucose derived from carbohydrates we wouldn't have the energy to move, breathe, talk, or think. We also need enormous amounts of energy to run the complicated mechanisms at work inside the body. For instance, absorbing and moving nutrients around the body takes energy, as does tissue repair and maintenance of other subtle systems that run our bodies. If our brain cells receive an inadequate supply of glucose, it will lead to confusion, hallucination, coma and even death. It is therefore critical that we receive an adequate amount of carbohydrate in our diet.

CHEMISTRY

There are two kinds of carbohydrates—sugars and complex carbohydrates. Sugars are made up of only one or two molecules and taste sweet. Complex carbohydrates, such as starches, are complicated structures comprised of many sugar molecules and do not taste sweet.

Plants use energy derived from the sun to form carbon dioxide and water into sugars. Eventually these sugars are joined into complex carbohydrates such as starches and cellulose. When we eat the plants the carbohydrates are broken down in our cells and release the energy they derived from the sun. In this sense, we run on solar energy.

There are many kinds of sugar but only glucose can be used by the body. This diagram of glucose will give you an idea of what a sugar molecule looks like.

Some sugars exist as single sugar units and are called monosaccharides. Others exist as double sugars and are called disaccharides. Sucrose—table sugar—is composed of two monosaccharides: glucose and fructose. Lactose—milk sugar—is composed of galactose and glucose. Maltose—sugar liberated by the breakdown of starches—is composed of two molecules of glucose.

The body must break disaccharides down into single sugar units and change them to glucose before they can be utilized. Monosaccharides are also called simple sugars.

63

Glucose

Disaccharides   Monosaccharides

Sucrose   =   Glucose   +   Fructose

Lactose   =   Galactose   +   Glucose

Maltose   =   Glucose   +   Glucose

When many sugars are joined together into polysaccharides, they are referred to as complex carbohydrates. Cellulose, the fibrous part of plants, and starch are examples of complex carbohydrates. Although both are composed of glucose molecules, they are joined together in a different manner. For this reason, cellulose and some other kinds of fiber cannot be digested by human enzymes. Cattle and other ruminants, however, can derive most of their calories from cellulose because their intestines are inhabited by bacteria which produce cellulose-digesting enzymes.

WHAT HAPPENS TO CARBOHYDRATE IN THE BODY

Although all carbohydrates are comprised of the same building blocks, the effect of sugars and complex carbohydrates on the body is quite different. Sugars enter the blood stream quickly. Complex carbohydrates, however, are broken down gradually into progressively shorter saccharide pieces with the aid of digestive enzymes in the mouth, small intestine and pancreas. Eventually they end up as single sugar units, are absorbed in the first three feet of the intestine and are carried by the portal vein to the liver. In the liver all sugars become glucose. Some of it is converted to glycogen, the form in which carbohydrate is stored. Glycogen is stored in the liver until needed and then will be broken down again to glucose. Sugar not converted to glycogen enters the bloodstream.

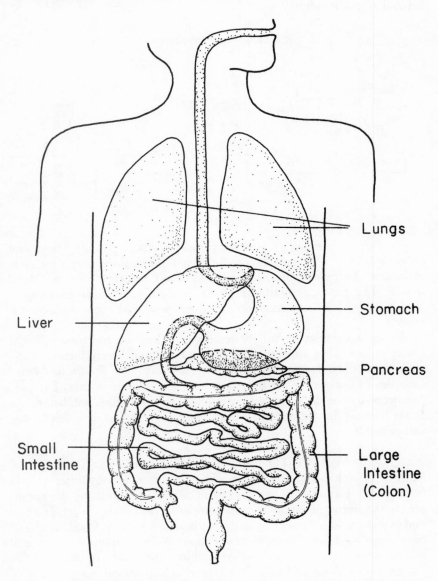

Lungs

Stomach

Liver

Pancreas

Small
Intestine

Large
Intestine
(Colon)

When blood reaches the pancreas, this organ is activated by the glucose, stimulating it to release insulin. Insulin is a hormone that enables glucose molecules in the blood to enter the body's cells. In the cells part of the glucose is burned (oxidized) to produce energy giving off carbon dioxide and water as waste products. A small amount of glucose is converted to glycogen and stored in muscle cells. The remaining glucose is converted to fat and stored in adipose tissues.

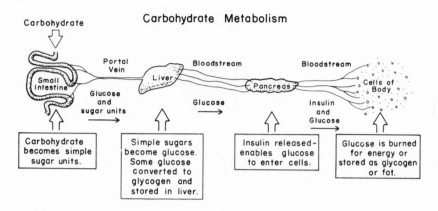

Carbohydrate Metabolism

With starches, which are complex carbohydrates, sugar enters the blood slowly and at an even rate. It takes quite a while to break down the large molecules. Therefore, glucose is produced and absorbed into the blood slowly. The pancreas is stimulated to produce only small amounts of insulin. This is the ideal situation, glucose is produced and utilized as it is needed.

We need complex carbohydrates because they are the most efficient source of fuel. They are completely utilized without the production of the toxic by-products formed from proteins and fats. (See *Protein and Fats*.) Complex carbohydrates are necessary for the utilization of fats. They are also necessary for the conservation of body protein, which will be broken down for fuel in the absence of sufficient carbohydrate to supply our energy needs.

WHAT TO EAT—WHAT TO AVOID

Most of the calories in our diet should come from carbohydrates, mainly from grains. Twenty-two percent of the calories consumed by Americans are in the form of complex carbohydrates. However, epidemiological studies show at least 75% of the calories consumed in Third World countries come from complex carbohydrates. People in these countries eat mostly grains, some legumes and root vegetables, and fruits in season. The Tarahumara Indians in Chihuahua, Mexico, for example, derive 90% of their calories from corn and beans. They are an extremely robust and healthy people.

People who adhere to a diet high in complex carbohydrates are almost free from cardiovascular disease, cancer, obesity, and diabetes. The best way to prevent and control these diseases is through diet—by increasing the amount of complex carbohydrates we eat, particularly grains.

Let me stress grains should be whole. We should avoid processed and refined grains because the fiber and most of the micro-nutrients have been removed.

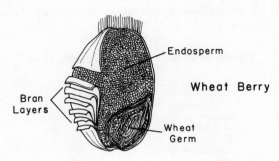

The outer coat of wheat and other grains is called the bran. It contains vitamins, minerals, proteins, and fiber. The fiber is brown and gives the color to whole grain flour. The inner part of the grain is the endosperm, the only part left after refining. It contains a small amount of protein, almost no vitamins or minerals, and a large quantity of starch. The germ or embryo from which the new plant sprouts is at the base of the grain. It is one of the richest known sources of vitamins B and E, and also contains proteins and vegetable oils.

Whole grains should accompany every meal. We can eat these grains in the form of cereal, pasta, or breads. Bread is no longer the staff of life in America, but should be. Good whole grain breads have appeared on the market again. It is also easy to make your own. (See *Foods*) Spaghetti and all kinds of pasta made with whole grains are available, but in some areas they can be obtained only in health food stores. Brown rice and barley are delicious, and you can add them to soups or stews. Experiment with all the grains until you find your favorites.

For breakfast, cook any whole grain cereal. If a ready-to-eat cereal is used, be sure you choose a variety made of whole grains. However convenient, these cereals should not be eaten routinely since they are low in essential amino acids and vitamins. Almost all the ready-to-eat cereals are made with refined flour, either wheat or corn. Most of the fiber, almost all the vitamins and minerals, and some of the essential amino acids have been destroyed or removed and few of the nutrients added back.

In order to prevent nutrient deficiency, refined American bread, ready-to-eat breakfast cereals and flour are now enriched with vitamins A, C and D and 5 of the B vitamins—thiamin, riboflavin, pyridoxine, niacin and folic acid. However, since the B vitamins work together, adding only some of them tends to cause a deficiency in the others. The B vitamins not replaced include PABA, inositol, choline and pantothenic acid. Also, almost all the vitamin E is removed.

Although minerals are also essential for the metabolism of carbohydrates, they are usually not added to carbohydrate foods depleted by refining. Iron is always replaced, and occasionally calcium. According to Dr. Henry Schroeder, the following percentages of the original mineral content remain after refining:

Percent of Minerals Remaining After Refining

Chromium	13
Manganese	9
Cobalt	30
Copper	10–30
Zinc	17
Molybdenum	50
Magnesium	17

(See *Vitamins* and *Minerals* for the effects on our health of the removal of nutrients.)

Sugars of all kinds, except those that are an integral part of whole, natural, unrefined foods should be avoided. The worst is refined white sugar. It should not be added to foods or used in food preparation at home. Foods commercially prepared contain large amounts of sugar and should be avoided. Even such natural sugars as honey contribute to the diseases discussed at the end of this chapter. The relative merits of various sugars and foods that contain them are discussed in the *Foods* chapter.

DISEASES OF SUGAR OVERCONSUMPTION

Replacing complex carbohydrates in the diet with sugar sets the scene for the onset of many diseases and pre-disease conditions.

Hypoglycemia: Our bodies have evolved to run on fuel in the form of complex carbohydrates. When we eat them, energy is produced slowly and the body can maintain fairly constant levels of blood sugar. This is not the case, however, with simple carbohydrates. The body tries to maintain even levels of glucose and when we consume sweets, large amounts of glucose are absorbed into the bloodstream all at once. This stimulates the pancreas to produce a large amount of insulin which quickly lowers the blood's level of glucose to below normal. This is hypoglycemia, or low blood sugar.

Several hormones act to raise the sugar and lower the insulin in the blood. Adrenaline is one of them. It is released in stressful situations to help us cope. Among other things, it acts to make sugar available for the production of energy to meet emergency situations. When hypoglycemia causes the release of adrenaline we have many of the same symptoms we have when we are angry, frightened, or upset. The heart beats faster, we get shaky, we perspire, and get weak or depressed. After a while the adrenaline will cause an increase in blood sugar by precipitating a breakdown of the liver's supply of glycogen to glucose. We stop secreting adrenaline and then feel better. If we eat sweets when the blood sugar is low, the cycle will be repeated.

A sudden dumping of glucose in the blood sets up an emergency situation the body must cope with. If these emergency situations happen frequently, repeated and exaggerated elevations and depressions of blood sugar will occur. The pancreas is stressed and could work less efficiently after a time. This is one reason why symptoms of hypoglycemia are commonly seen before the onset of diabetes.

Diabetes: High blood sugar—diabetes—is a disease characterized by the inability to metabolize carbohydrates, protein and fat properly. Dr. Ira Laufer of the New York Diabetes Association, states that diabetes is a disease of affluence and is related to food intake. Historically, poor societies have eaten diets high in complex carbohydrates because they cost less. Complex carbohydrates in their natural state are broken down to glucose slowly. Sucrose—table sugar—is a highly concentrated and unnatural food. It is made by processing natural foods, beets and sugar cane, until nothing is left but pure double sugars. After processing, nothing inhibits its immediate entry into the bloodstream. Now that sugar is plentiful and cheap, 10 million people in America suffer from diabetes and the number is increasing at the rate of 6% a year. Diabetes is the third leading cause of death in the United States. Two percent of the population of Western countries suffer from at least a mild form of the disease. In the early part of the nineteenth century the per capita use of sugar was less than 10 lb. per year. Now it is more than 130 lb. a year.

Many factors are involved in the cause of diabetes—stress, heredity, certain viral infections that damage the pancreas, obesity, insufficient physical activity, and excessive fat and sugar consumption. However, only nutritional factors are within the scope of this book.

Habitual indulging in large amounts of sugar can stress the pancreas by constant demands for massive secretions of insulin, diminishing its ability to react efficiently. Rats fed large amounts of sugar develop abnormalities of the pancreas and impaired ability to metabolize carbohydrates.

Tolbutamide is a drug used to treat diabetes. It lowers blood sugar by stimulating the pancreas to produce more insulin. If the pancreas is damaged, the drug will not be able to cause as great a rise in insulin as it will if the pancreas is healthy. Rats fed a high sugar diet for several weeks did not have as great a depression of blood sugar after tolbutamide therapy as did rats fed on a high starch diet. This proved a diet high in sugar will eventually cause exhaustion of the part of the pancreas responsible for insulin production.

No wonder that a high sugar diet is so strongly implicated as one of the contributing factors in the development of diabetes. Dr. Jean Mayer, one of our foremost nutritionists, says diet is the main cause of diabetes and the most important part of treatment.

There is much epidemiological evidence that a high sugar diet causes diabetes, especially the adult-onset type. In a recent comparative study of two American Indian tribes, the greater intake of sucrose by one tribe was hypothesized to be responsible for their significantly higher blood glucose levels.

Dr. G. D. Campbell found a much higher incidence of diabetes among the Indians living in Natal, South Africa, than among their relatives still living in India. The average sugar consumption in Natal is 110 lb. a year; in India it is 12-15 lb. The wealthier Indians in Natal who can afford a more highly refined diet, have a higher incidence of diabetes than have the poor. While overconsumption of simple carbohydrates is believed by some researchers to be one of the causative factors in the development of diabetes, a diet high in unrefined complex carbohydrates has been found effective in its treatment. In addition, it helps prevent the cardiovascular complications usually accompanying the disease.

Liver Disease: The pancreas is not the only organ to suffer from overindulgence in sugar. The liver is also involved in metabolic processes that maintain the normal blood levels of sugar and it, too, can suffer the consequences of overconsumption. A healthy liver has all it can do to handle small quantities of sugar in its natural form.

As stated earlier, when excessive sugar is eaten, the level of blood sugar becomes temporarily too high. In the attempt to lower it, the liver converts some of the glucose into glycogen. Glycogen is a very large, complex and compact polysaccharide molecule sometimes referred to as animal starch. The liver can only store a certain amount of glucose in this form, however, and it converts the rest to fatty acids. This causes fat to accumulate in the liver rapidly leading to an increase in the number of liver cells (hyperplasia) and an increase in the size of the cells (hypertrophy).

Adrenal Disease: The body lowers blood sugar by secreting insulin. Excessive lowering of blood sugar by insulin causes a counter reaction, the secretion of adrenaline. Adrenaline is secreted in emergencies and causes rapid beating of the heart, sweating, paleness, and a feeling of anxiety. A diet high in sugar causes the adrenal gland to secrete more adrenaline from the inner part of the gland and more adrenocortical hormones from the

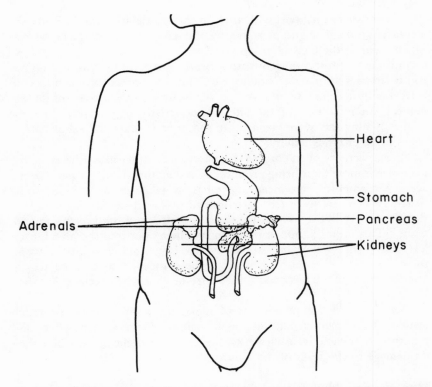

Heart

Stomach

Pancreas

Adrenals

Kidneys

outer part of the gland. This stress can lead to hypertrophy and hyperplasia in this gland also.

Atherosclerosis: Sugar is implicated by some researchers in atherosclerosis. When the blood sugar level is elevated, the liver converts glucose to fatty acids. Consuming too much sugar will, therefore, result in increased triglycerides—fats—in the blood, and this is a contributing factor in the development of atherosclerosis. When you eat complex carbohydrates, the glucose enters the blood slowly and the formation of fats is not necessary to maintain blood glucose within normal limits.

Dr. A. M. Cohen did studies on Yemenites in Jerusalem. He found little heart disease among the immigrants but it was common among those who had been in Israel for 20 years. Both groups ate a high-fat diet, but the immigrants had been eating much less sugar in the Yemen. Metabolic studies show that sugar is related to increases in blood triglycerides more than any other food.

John Yudkin, Professor of Nutrition and Dietetics at the University of London, is of the opinion that the consumption of sugar is an important factor in the causation of heart attacks and atherosclerosis in the leg arteries. In a study, he used three groups of subjects. One group consisted of patients who had recently suffered their first heart attack; the second group consisted of patients with artery disease in the leg, and the third was a control group. The groups with arterial disease consumed nearly twice as much sugar as the control group.

In order to protect ourselves from heart disease we must be careful not to eat fatty foods or sugar. Studies were done on one of the enzymes concerned with fat synthesis and storage. An increase in the activity of this enzyme is an indication of the fat-forming activity of the liver. In these studies, young rats were given sugar and after 10 days they showed five times more enzyme activity.

Greater activity of an enzyme complex called fatty acid synthetase in the liver means more fat is being produced. On the other hand, greater enzyme activity in adipose tissue means more fats are taken from the blood to be stored. When rats were fed sugar instead of starch for 30 days the synthetase activity in the liver doubled yet dropped to a third in the adipose tissues. This means although more fat was being put into the blood, even less than usual was being stored. Much larger amounts of fat were, therefore, in the circulatory system where they cause damage to the arteries. Sugar in the diet causes these enzyme changes to occur in less than 24 hours.

When we eat a large amount of sugar, the body secretes too much insulin. Subsequently anti-insulin hormones such as adrenaline and pituitrin are released, causing elevated levels of fats in the blood where they do damage to the walls of the arteries.

Hypertension (High Blood Pressure): The results of recent research show sucrose plays a role in the development of hypertension in rats and monkeys. Salt intake influences blood pressure to a greater extent, but sucrose affects the amount of salt retained in the body. An increase in blood pressure is caused by only moderate amounts of sucrose. Large amounts can cause kidney damage.

Hyperactivity: Dr. Lendon H. Smith explains why 20–30% of school children have learning problems. The upper brain, the cerebral cortex, which is the seat of cognitive skills is extremely dependent on adequate levels of blood glucose. When these levels sink too low, children cannot function normally; they are dietary hyperactives.

Sugar can have a stimulating effect on the hyperactive child. These children are often intelligent but they have behavior and learning problems. Symptoms include difficulty in learning to read, spell and write, lack of coordination, poor visual skills, a short attention span, hyperactivity, and confused eye-hand preference. Some hyperactive children suffer from poor nutrition and hypoglycemia. Because eating sugar will cause low blood sugar, the efficiency and learning ability of the brain is lowered. Cola beverages are harmful because they contain large amounts of sugar and the stimulant caffeine.

Ulcers: Dr. John Yudkin studied sugar as an irritant to the linings of the esophagus, stomach and duodenum. Gastric analysis of young men showed the acidity of gastric juices increased by about 20% and enzyme activity increased almost three-fold when they were given sugar. This implicates sugar as a factor in indigestion as well as gastric and duodenal ulcers.

Sugar can also be a contributing factor in ulcers because of its osmotic effect. Certain substances draw water to themselves from their surroundings. For instance, if you sprinkle salt on cabbage, it will wilt and water will be extracted. Sugar also has a high osmotic effect, although to a lesser degree. Sprinkle sugar on fruit and the juices will be extracted to form a sweet syrup. The same happens in the stomach and intestines. Sugar molecules are small and numerous and they draw water from the cells lining the stomach and intestine. Starch molecules are larger and fewer in number and have less tendency to draw water to themselves. Sugar molecules exert such a high osmotic pressure they can prevent the growth of bacteria which is why sugar is used as a preservative. This action can be very irritating to sensitive cells.

Tooth Decay: Unlike other diseases caused by our diet, tooth decay is an infectious rather than a degenerative disease. There are bacteria in the plaque coating our teeth. When a lot of sugar, especially sucrose, is eaten the bacteria produce acid which causes tooth decay. During both World Wars, when sugar was scarce in Europe, the incidence of tooth decay in children sharply dropped.

Obesity: Eating too much sugar will cause excessive amounts of insulin to be secreted, causing the body to turn the sugar into fat rather than energy. Insulin also brings about a lowering of blood sugar. The result is an extreme feeling of hunger that can lead to overeating. People attempting to lose weight should avoid all sugar.

We may never know all the harm done to the body from our large sugar intake, but it is obvious we should cut down on its consumption. You may wonder how sugar could cause so many diseases. Bear in mind we are not dealing with an ordinary food. Sugar enters the system faster than most drugs and has effects similar to many potent medications. It enters the system so rapidly it causes hormonal changes. The results are far reaching and extremely dangerous.

There are two different kinds of carbohydrates—simple and complex. They react very differently in the body and we cannot speak of the effect of carbohydrates unless we specify which one we mean. The words carbohy-drate and starch have a bad connotation to most people. We must remember starch is a complex carbohydrate and is very healthful in its unrefined state.

The sugar and candy industries have advertised so much that we now aassociate their products with "quick energy." The public thinks of this as nutritionally desirable. There is no physiological need for sugar, and it is strongly implicated in most of the diseases afflicting the civilized world. All foods contain energy. Sugar is advertised as possessing energy because that is all it contains.

Chapter 5

FATS AND OTHER LIPIDS

Lipids (fats and fat-like substances) are a necessary part of the diet and serve many functions in the body. One of the most important is the storage of energy in the fat cells. Energy can be stored in a much more concentrated form as fat, and most of an animal's energy is stored that way. Plants, being stationary, do not need energy in such a concentrated form, and therefore store their energy as starch. Only the seeds of plants store most of their energy as fat. This is because they are very small, yet must supply the new plant life with energy as it develops.

Lipids also serve as structural components of membranes. They are the most important part of the cell wall; because of their insolubility in water, they help control which substances leave and enter the cell.

CHEMISTRY

Lipids are fats and fat-like substances that include fats, fatty acids, cholesterol, lipoproteins, and phospholipids. Like carbohydrates, they are composed of carbon, hydrogen and oxygen. However, they contain these elements in different proportions. In carbohydrates there are 10 parts of carbon and 20 parts of hydrogen to 10 parts of oxygen, while in fats the same amounts of carbon and hydrogen are combined with only 1 part of oxygen.

Carbohydrate: $C_{10}H_{20}O_{10}$—4 calories/gram
Fat: $C_{10}H_{20}O_1$—9 calories/gram

Because fats contain much less oxygen, they are more highly concentrated fuels. A much higher percentage of the fat molecule can be burned (combined with oxygen) to produce energy, which is why there are 9 calories in each gram of fat that we eat and only 4 in each gram of carbohydrate.

Fatty acids are long carbon chains. Hydrogen is attached to the carbon atoms, except for the one on the end of the chain which is attached to oxygen.

$$\left(C \overset{\displaystyle O}{\underset{\displaystyle OH}{\diagup}} \right)$$

This part of the molecule is slightly acid; that is why they are called fatty *acids*.

Fatty acids can be saturated or unsaturated. Those that are not saturated can be either mono - or polyunsaturated.

```
    H  H  H  H  H  H  H  H  H  H  H  H  H  H  H  H  H  H
    |  |  |  |  |  |  |  |  |  |  |  |  |  |  |  |  |  |    O
 H- C- C- C- C- C- C- C- C- C- C- C- C- C- C- C- C- C- C ∥
    |  |  |  |  |  |  |  |  |  |  |  |  |  |  |  |  |  |    OH
    H  H  H  H  H  H  H  H  H  H  H  H  H  H  H  H  H  H
```

Stearic Acid - Example of a Saturated Fatty Acid

An example of a fatty acid is stearic acid (shown above) which is abundant in animal tissues. This is called a *saturated* fatty acid because all the carbon atoms are bonded to hydrogen atoms. In other words, its carbon atoms are saturated with hydrogen atoms.

Unsaturated fatty acids lack at least one pair of hydrogen atoms. That means that two of the carbon atoms have only one hydrogen atom attached to each. Oleic acid is a monounsaturated fatty acid because only one pair of hydrogen atoms is missing.

```
    H  H  H  H  H  H  H  H  H  H  H  H  H  H  H  H  H  H
    |  |  |  |  |  |  |  |     |  |  |  |  |  |  |  |  |    O
 H- C- C- C- C- C- C- C- C- C= C- C- C- C- C- C- C- C- C ∥
    |  |  |  |  |  |  |  |     |  |  |  |  |  |  |  |  |    OH
    H  H  H  H  H  H  H  H     H  H  H  H  H  H  H  H
```

Oleic Acid - Example of a Monounsaturated Fatty Acid

Linoleic acid is an example of a polyunsaturated acid. More than one pair of hydrogen atoms is missing. Linoleic is called by some researchers the only essential fatty acid. Others consider linolenic essential also.

```
    H  H  H  H  H  H  H  H  H  H  H  H  H  H  H  H  H  H
    |  |  |  |  |     |  |     |  |  |  |  |  |  |  |  |    O
 H- C- C- C- C- C- C= C- C- C= C- C- C- C- C- C- C- C- C ∥
    |  |  |  |  |     |        |  |  |  |  |  |  |  |  |    OH
    H  H  H  H  H     H        H  H  H  H  H  H  H  H
```

Linoleic Acid - Example of a Polyunsaturated Fatty Acid

Triglyceride is another name for fat or oil. The difference between fats and oils is that fats are solid at room temperature while oils are fluid. Those that tend to be solid usually contain more saturated fatty acids. A triglyceride is composed of three fatty acids and glycerol which is a small three-carbon molecule.

```
┌───┬──────────────────────────────────┐
│ G │        FATTY   ACID              │
│ L ├──────────────────────────────────┤
│ Y │                                  │
│ C │        FATTY   ACID              │
│ E ├──────────────────────────────────┤
│ R │                                  │
│ O │        FATTY   ACID              │
│ L │                                  │
└───┴──────────────────────────────────┘
```

Triglyceride   or   Fat   Molecule

If glycerol has only one fatty acid attached, it is called a monoglyceride. With two fatty acids it is a diglyceride. If you read grocery labels you have seen the terms mono- and diglycerides. They can be made synthetically and are added to foods since they help prevent separation. In the body, mono- and diglycerides are either triglycerides being broken down into fatty acids to be used for energy or in the process of being built up into triglycerides to be stored. Therefore, most glycerides in the body are in the form of triglycerides.

Just as single sugars are the building blocks of carbohydrates, fatty acids are the building blocks of fats (triglycerides). However, there are relatively few kinds of monosaccharides or simple sugars, while over 70 different fatty acids have been found in our cells and tissues. The main differences between the fatty acids are the length of the carbon chains— whether they are saturated or have hydrogen pairs missing—and the location of the missing pairs of hydrogen.

The term saturated fats or unsaturated fats refers to whether or not the fatty acids of which they are composed are saturated with hydrogen.

WHAT HAPPENS TO LIPIDS IN THE BODY

Fats are insoluble in water and form large globules which are difficult to break down. To facilitate digestion, bile, secreted by the liver and stored in the gall bladder, is discharged into the small intestine. Bile acts as an emulsifier, allowing fat globules to be dispersed by the churning action in the intestine. This causes a greater surface area of the fats to be exposed to the digestive enzymes. They are broken down into fatty acids and glycerol, absorbed into the cells of the intestine and re-formed into molecules of fat. Microscopic globules of fat (chylomicrons) accumulate in the intestinal cells and turn the walls of the intestine a whitish color. Chylomicrons enter the lymphatic system and if enough fatty food has been eaten, turn the lymph white. Fat is carried by the lymph to the blood which becomes viscous and milky white when it receives large amounts.

When fats enter the cells, they are again broken apart into glycerol and fatty acids. Two molecules of glycerol, each containing three carbon atoms, can then be used to form one molecule of glucose, containing six carbons. Or the glycerol can be broken down to produce energy. Most of the fat molecule is composed of large fatty acid molecules. Although this part of the molecule cannot be converted to sugar, it can be burned and is the source of most of the energy of fats.

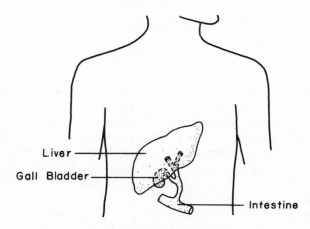

Liver
Gall Bladder
Intestine

Organs of Fat Digestion

WHAT TO EAT—WHAT TO AVOID

Although fats are of the utmost importance, we need them only in small amounts. In excess, they can cause a great deal of harm.

In order to decrease your intake of fats, avoid red meat and full-fat dairy products. Use skim milk and dairy products made from skim milk. Substitute fish and poultry for red meat. Avoid nuts and nut butters.

Oils and oil products should be avoided. They are high in polyunsaturated fats which are oxidized to harmful substances causing, among other things, heart disease, cancer and premature aging. Whole foods containing polyunsaturated fats also contain vitamin E and selenium which inhibit the oxidation of fats. Extracted oils contain little or no antioxidants and our excessive consumption of oils increases the need for them.

Feeding infants, especially the premature, formulas with a high content of polyunsaturated fatty acids can result in a low vitamin E/fatty acid ratio, causing anemia. This can be corrected with vitamin E supplementation. It can be prevented by feeding a formula lower in polyunsaturated fatty acids.

It is best to obtain vitamin E from the foods we eat. However, we cannot get enough in this manner if we continue using large amounts of vegetable oils on salads, in baking, in mayonnaise, in artificial creamers and in spreads. The *Foods* chapter tells you how to avoid the use of oils and products made from them in your cooking. Additional reasons for avoiding the use of margarine is discussed in the same chapter. We should obtain fats in our diet from whole foods rather than extracting them. Ample amounts are provided in vegetables, grains, and legumes.

We do not need to eat foods that contain all the different kinds of fatty acids. The body can convert one type to the other with the exception of linoleic and possibly linolenic acid. Because our bodies cannot make linoleic acid, it is called the essential fatty acid and we must obtain it from our food. Linoleic acid must account for one percent of an adult's caloric intake. We can easily obtain this amount when whole foods predominate in the diet.

In addition to oils, there is another substance which should be avoided in its extracted form. It is lecithin, which has been a subject of much interest in the press during the last several years. It is a phospholipid whose molecule is very similar to fat molecules. Like fats, it is composed of glycerol and fatty acids, but it contains only two instead of three fatty acids. In place of the third fatty acid, it contains a molecule of phosphate and a molecule of choline. Because the phospholipids are both water and fat soluble they function well as emulsifying agents; they cause fats to be dispersed in the form of minute globules. For this reason, lecithin is used commercially in foods such as mayonnaise, margarine, ice cream, and bakery products. It also has many uses in industry. In the body, it changes large fat particles into smaller ones, and it also increases the amount of fat absorption from the intestine.

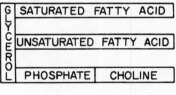

Fat   Lecithin

Advocates have claimed that lecithin lowers blood cholesterol. It is broken down in the same manner as fats. Any cholesterol-lowering effect is caused by the same mechanisms that cause unsaturated fats to lower the cholesterol in the blood. In other words, it may be ridding the blood of cholesterol by driving it right into the walls of your arteries. It can also increase the level of blood cholesterol, especially in those people who have low cholesterol.

Lecithin is produced in the liver. It is also found in grains and legumes and all other unrefined foods containing oil. Choline is part of the lecithin molecule and the body can use it to make lecithin. Choline is sometimes considered a member of the vitamin B family and it is found in the same foods as the B vitamins. Rats fed choline-deficient diets by Canadian researchers died from abnormalities of the arteries. This research shows that the body has a need for choline. However, when lecithin is broken down by the body, most of the molecule will be used as a fat. Excessive amounts will cause the same problems caused by consuming too much fat.

It is unnecessary to worry about getting sufficient lecithin or choline as they are found in many unrefined foods. Lecithin is an energy-rich substance containing 7 calories per gram. Excessive consumption in the form of supplementation should be avoided.

DISEASES OF LIPID OVERCONSUMPTION

As previously stated, lipids are an absolute necessity but only in small amounts. In fact, if more than moderate amounts are ingested, they will cause problems.

Atherosclerosis: Cardiovascular disease is the leading cause of death in the United States, affecting nearly 29 million people. There is much greater incidence of this disease in our country than in less developed countries. The main cause of heart disease is a diet too high in fats.

A diet high in fats encourages the body to make too much cholesterol. Cholesterol is a lipid but it is not a fat. This lipid was first isolated from humans in the form of gallstones. It is solid and wax-like and insoluble in the blood, except when in combination with lipoproteins.

Cholesterol serves many important functions. It is a part of cell walls. It is a precursor of bile acids, vitamin D, and many steroid hormones, including the adrenal and sex hormones. It is also a necessary part of the lipoproteins which allow lipids to be soluble in the blood. Although cholesterol is vital, there is no need to include it in the diet since it is produced in ample amounts by the body. Cholesterol can be quite harmful if excessive amounts are consumed. Epidemiological studies have proven that the intake of dietary cholesterol correlates with the incidence of heart disease. Many factors increase the risk of death attributable to atherosclerosis, but the greatest risk factor of all is a high concentration of cholesterol in the blood.

Cholesterol is found in all foods from animal sources but is not found in foods from plant sources. It is in all meat, especially organ meats, egg yolks, and dairy products. It is formed in excessive amounts by the body when we consume large amounts of fat.

Lipids are insoluble in water and blood. In order to be transported in the blood, they become attached to proteins which are water soluble. This combined form of lipid and protein is called a lipoprotein. If we eat too much oily or fatty food, causing the liver to manufacture more cholesterol, there will be too much of it to be carried in the lipoprotein. Cholesterol falls off the lipoproteins rather easily, especially in the arteries where the pressure is high and the substances in the blood are bumped about roughly. Cholesterol which falls off is not soluble in the blood and drops to the vessel wall where it is used in the building of arterial plaques. Plaques are like hard sores composed of cholesterol, fats, fibrous tissue, calcium, and other substances. They cause a narrowing of the artery and inhibit the flow of blood.

The walls of arteries constantly sustain minor injuries. Cells exposed by the injury ingest fats and cholesterol. If excessive amounts of these lipids are in the blood, the cells proliferate. They become engorged and begin to look like "foam" cells, which is what they are called. If enough lipids are ingested, the cells burst. The body will then encapsulate the area in fibrous tissue. The artery walls become hard and lose their elasticity making it easier for them to sustain further injury. Although the fibrous tissue laid down serves as a protection from the lipid-laden blood in the artery, small blood vessels that feed the cells of the artery wall continue supplying cholesterol to the foam cells. More of these cells will burst and new ones will continue to be made until the entire plaque bursts. Pieces of debris may be released into the blood stream. Now clots may form around the sores which become lodging places for more cholesterol. As the build-up increases, the size of the blood vessel decreases. Sometimes the artery becomes completely closed, preventing blood from reaching the tissues. Sometimes clots formed on the plaques or pieces of debris break loose and are carried by the blood to a smaller vessel causing it to become blocked.

Normal and Occluded Artery

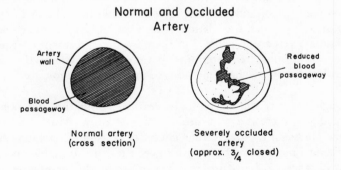

Artery wall

Reduced blood passageway

Blood passageway

Normal artery (cross section)

Severely occluded artery (approx. 3/4 closed)

The hardening and narrowing of the arteries is called atherosclerosis. In some people it can be reversed by a diet low in lipids. It is best to make dietary changes when young, as reversal is more effective in the early stages of disease.

Some people replace saturated fats in their diet with vegetable oils. They believe only saturated fats cause atherosclerosis and unsaturated fats actually afford them protection from it. About twenty years ago, it was found that when people consumed rather large quantities of unsaturated fats in the form of extracted vegetable oils, the level of cholesterol in their blood sometimes was lowered. During the following years, there was much discussion of the ratio of polyunsaturated oils to that of saturated fats in the diet. The consumption of large amounts of vegetable oils was advocated; it was suggested that polyunsaturated and saturated oils should be consumed in a ratio of 1.5 to 1. Now, however, it has been found that people living in areas low in atherosclerosis consume about equal amounts of saturated and polyunsaturated oils. It has been discovered that a low level of blood cholesterol is not necessarily a good indication of the health of the arteries.It is hypothesized now that unsaturated fats cause the cholesterol to be redistributed from the blood to the tissues. And, it is suspected that increasing the amount of unsaturated fat in the diet causes the cholesterol to be deposited directly into the arterial walls.

In studies on humans polyunsaturated fats sometimes cause a decrease in plasma cholesterol but the response varies from person to person. In some people a lowering of the plasma cholesterol is accompanied by an increased excretion of cholesterol or its breakdown products in the feces, but in some people this is not the case.

At the Rockefeller University, studies led by Edward H. Ahrens, demonstrated that when humans are fed unsaturated fats, the decrease in blood cholesterol is frequently due to the redistribution of cholesterol from the blood into the tissues. Instead of being carried in the blood, the cholesterol falls off the lipoproteins and is taken up by the tissues, especially the arteries.

Polyunsaturated fats change the metabolism of lipids, but although there have been many studies in this area, no one knows how the metabolism is changed. There is much speculation as to what happens to the cholesterol when plasma levels are lowered, but there is little agreement on the question. It is impossible to determine with certainty where the missing cholesterol goes until we have methods to measure the cholesterol in body tissues.

Although there is still much to be learned about the metabolism of unsaturated fats, there is a great deal that we *do* know. Much research has been done lately on the deleterious effects of consuming polyunsaturated fats. These fats readily combine with oxygen to form unstable and highly reactive substances. Polyunsaturated lipids make up the membranes of tiny cell parts whose functions are similar to those of the body's organs. In the presence of oxygen, the lipids of these membranes can become free radicals that can react with and damage or destroy proteins. They cause proteins to undergo changes such as polymerization where they form extremely large, heavy, and inflexible molecules. This results in a loss of elasticity in tissues.

The formation of these large molecules causes premature aging of the major protein of connective tissue, cartilage, and bone and premature aging of the major connective tissue of such elastic structures as the large blood vessels. Free radicals formed by the oxidation of polyunsaturated oils join with two protein molecules in a process called cross-linking. Cross-linking contributes to the aging process by causing a loss of elasticity in the tissues of the body, an action quite obvious in skin tissue. It also results in the loss of elasticity in arterial walls causing tiny cracks that can lead to atherosclerosis.

Heart Attack: The heart muscle is supplied with blood by the coronary arteries. If a piece of plaque or a clot breaks loose it can become lodged in the opening of a small or damaged vessel completely blocking it and shutting off the blood supply to that area. If this happens in a heart vessel, it results in a heart attack or myocardial infarction. This may result in death. A person may survive a heart attack, but the part of the heart that loses its blood supply will die. When part of the heart muscle is dead, the heart no longer functions properly especially when we engage in physical activities.

Although a cardiac vessel does not become completely occluded, it can become dangerously narrow. When we engage in strenuous exercise under these circumstances, the part of the heart receiving an insufficient supply of blood will contract at the wrong time. The heart will have an irregular rhythm. Such an arrhythmia can result in fibrillation: an extremely rapid, shallow, and inefficient beating of the heart that does not allow the heart to empty completely nor move the blood strongly enough. The cells of the body become starved for oxygen. If allowed to continue, fibrillation results in death, and it is too late to cut down on our intake of fats.

Many heart attacks occur upon exertion, or after a heavy meal. The fats in the meal make it difficult for the cells of the body, including heart cells, to receive sufficient oxygen.

After eating a high fat meal, the extra fat in the blood coats the red cells making them sticky. These red cells carry oxygen to the body's other cells, but to do so they must pass through the capillaries, the smallest of the blood vessels. Since these round, flat cells are almost twice as big as the capillaries, they must bend over like a folded taco, one at a time, to squeeze through. When they stick together, they aren't flexible enough and they block the capillaries. The cells of the body including those in the heart become deprived of oxygen.

Red Cells and Capillaries

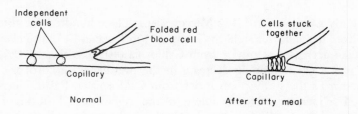

Independent cells

Folded red blood cell

Capillary

Normal

Cells stuck together

Capillary

After fatty meal

The peak of digestion occurs seven hours after eating. If a fatty meal is eaten in the evening, the fatty blood will move slowly through the arteries during sleep. This leads to the development of plaques and the formation of clots which can cause strokes.

During the Korean War a report was released by the Armed Forces Institute of Pathology. On autopsy examination of American, Chinese and Korean soldiers killed in action in Korea large plaques were seen in the coronary arteries of 50% of the Americans. Their average age was 22 years. In 10% of these soldiers, one of the three major coronary arteries was reduced more than 50%. However, there were no lipid deposits in the coronary arteries of the Chinese and Korean soldiers who normally consume no milk and only small amounts of eggs and meat.

Since then, there has been much research in this area. Many factors have been found to increase the risk of developing coronary disease. However, of all the risk factors, elevated levels of blood cholesterol increase the chances of developing coronary heart disease more than any of the others.

What can we do about these high levels of cholesterol? We can decrease the amount of cholesterol-containing foods we eat.

Early studies did not find a correlation between dietary and serum cholesterol since cholesterol was administered in a manner in which it could not be absorbed. Subsequent studies, however, clearly demonstrated the relationship between the amount of cholesterol we eat and the amount of cholesterol in the blood.

A large study on the autopsy findings of more than 31,000 men, women, and children in 15 countries found correlations between the fat intake, serum cholesterol levels, and the degree of hardening of the coronary vessels. Another large study on 12,000 men from 7 countries between the ages of 40–59 indicated the highest rates of cardiovascular disease existed in the United States and Finland; the lowest were in Japan. The rates correlated with the amount of cholesterol in the blood.

In order to disprove the idea that some populations suffer more from cardiovascular disease because of genetic differences, research has been performed comparing the diet and health of immigrants with that of their countrymen who have remained at home and adhered to the traditional diet.

A study was done on 1,372 Micronesians. Three hundred and fifteen of them lived in California, 628 in Guam, 271 in Rota and 158 in Palau. The fat intake decreased step-wise from California (40%) to Palau (20%), and there was a corresponding decrease in the prevalence of coronary heart disease across the study populations from California to Palau. There was progressive increase in blood cholesterol and triglycerides, histories of heart attacks, and certain EKG abnormalities from the traditional to the Westernized areas.

In another study migrant workers in our country had a cardiovascular death rate more similar to citizens of the United States than to people in the country of their birth.

Adolescents and even children in this country have shockingly high levels of serum cholesterol and are developing plaques in their young arteries. In man and other mammals the blood cholesterol is low at birth and increases rapidly during the first few months of life while the infant is nursing. However, cholesterol levels of people in developed countries continue to increase after weaning, whereas they decrease in people of undeveloped countries and in wild animals.

In view of these findings, I think the need for a change in the diet of Americans is obvious, including a change in the diet of children. Cholesterol levels above 220 greatly increase the risk of developing heart disease. A survey of Iowa teenagers revealed that the blood cholesterol in 15% of them was above this level. Studies show that adherence to a low fat diet results in a decrease in the amount of cholesterol in the blood.

There are people who believe there is no relationship between dietary fat and the incidence of heart disease based on the fact that mortality statistics for Eskimos do not list heart attacks as a major cause of death even though their fat intake is high. Several factors account for this. One reason they do not appear to have much heart disease is the fact that many Eskimos do not live beyond the age of 40. Among those who live longer, atherosclerotic disease is common. Another reason for the apparent low incidence of heart disease is inaccuracy in the death statistics.

Some people believe that it does not matter how much cholesterol is in the diet. They say that when you ingest more, your body makes less and when you eat less, your body makes more. Actually, cholesterol intake does not repress its synthesis in the body. At levels over 600 mg. cholesterol per day there is no increase in blood cholesterol because additional cholesterol is deposited in other tissues.

Articles about HDL in the blood protecting us against heart disease are appearing in newspapers and magazines. Physicians are testing for it with increasing frequency. HDL (high density lipoprotein) is one type of lipoprotein which carries the insoluble fats and cholesterol in the blood. It carries cholesterol to the liver and from there it is eliminated. LDL is another lipoprotein carrying fats and cholesterol. It carries cholesterol from the liver and is implicated in depositing cholesterol in the arteries. HDL, on the other hand, is believed to serve as a protection against atherosclerosis.

It has been found that people with higher levels of LDL tend to suffer from atherosclerosis. Elevated levels of LDL seem to constitute a risk factor for coronary heart disease just as do smoking, obesity, and high blood pressure. If the diet is low in fats, the liver will produce less LDL and increase the amount of HDL. On a low fat, highly unrefined diet, high in complex carbohydrates, the HDL will increase by the end of the second month. Exercise has the same effect. HDL levels are higher in those who exercise, in non-smokers, in those who are underweight, and in premenopausal females. Women in the age bracket where they are producing large amounts of female sex hormones are partially protected since these hormones affect the liver in its handling of fats. Women in the childbearing age, therefore, tend to produce less cholesterol and less LDL. Because of this fact, some physicians started treating their male patients who had suffered one or more heart attacks with estrogen, the female sex hormone. However, although this treatment did raise the level of HDL, it did not prevent further heart attacks.

Some researchers believe the level of the dangerous LDL is not as important as the total cholesterol/HDL and the LDL/HDL ratios. In other words, they think higher levels of HDL will partially protect against heart attack. In their opinion, high levels of HDL cholesterol are more important than the amount of LDL or total cholesterol.

Other researchers continue to feel that total cholesterol is the most important risk-determining factor. In any case, it is obvious that foods containing large amounts of fats (both saturated and unsaturated) and cholesterol must be avoided. If this type of food is avoided, both the "good" HDL will be increased and the "bad" LDL and total amount of cholesterol in the blood will be decreased. If this type of food is not avoided, we won't see a decrease in the epidemic incidence of coronary heart disease.

Angina Pectoris: Angina is chest pain or pain in the area of the left shoulder or arm caused by sclerosis (hardening) of the arteries that supply the heart itself. Many older people suffer from it. The vessels become narrowed to such an extent that the arteries are too constricted to allow an adequate supply of oxygen-bearing blood to the heart. This causes pain during exercise. Angina is not a disease but a symptom of cardiovascular disease.

Claudication: Claudication is a symptom of hardening of the blood vessels in the legs. When these vessels become narrowed, exercise causes a lack of oxygen to the leg muscles. This results in pain of the calves or feet and makes walking impossible. The condition can be so severe that a half a block is too far to walk without being stopped by pain.

Cancer: In populations consuming a high fat diet there is not only more heart disease, but an increased incidence of cancer. Dr. Ernst Wynder, a prominent researcher in the area of cancer and president of the American Health Foundation, states that the diet linked to atherosclerosis is also linked to cancer. Most cancer, according to Dr. Wynder, is caused by nutritional *excesses* and the incidence of this kind of cancer continues to increase.

The nutritional excess leading to cancer in industrialized countries is lipids—cholesterol and fats. Both saturated and unsaturated fats have been implicated. In fact, it is believed that unsaturated fats are more carcinogenic than saturated. Unsaturated fats easily become oxidized. When they do, they can damage our genetic material. When chromosomes are altered, it is called mutation. This is the same kind of mutation caused by radiation. Chromosomal changes are the direct cause of cancer. Experiments on rodents demonstrated the carcinogenic and life-shortening effects of a diet high in unsaturated fats as compared with a diet high in saturated fats.

Cancer of the colon is the most common cause of death due to cancer in the United States. Epidemiological studies show that the incidence of colon cancer correlates with the amount of fat in the diet. Steroids such as bile acids and cholesterol are broken down in the intestine by bacteria into substances that cause cancer. Excessive dietary fat causes an increase in the amount of these substances in the intestine. It also causes an increase in the number of the kind of bacteria that break them down. In addition, a high fat diet is, almost by definition, low in fiber which dilutes the concentration of carcinogens in the intestine.

People who migrate from areas where there is little risk of colon cancer, such as Japan, to areas of high risk, such as the United States, become as prone as we are to developing this type of cancer. Those people living in Japan who do have cancer of the colon tend to be wealthier and to eat a diet more similar to that eaten in Western countries. In Hawaii people eat more fat than in Japan but less than in the United States. Among Japanese who migrate to Hawaii, the incidence of cancer of the colon is between that of Japan and the United States.

The increase in dietary fat (especially unsaturated fat) correlates not only with colon cancer but with cancer of the breast, ovary, endometrium (lining of the uterus), prostate, rectum and of leukemia. Data concerning the diets eaten in different countries were collected by the United Nations in 1964. On examination of these data, a significant correlation was found between the consumption of fats and oils and the death rates from breast cancer.

As with colon cancer, the incidence of breast cancer in people of Japanese ancestry correlates with the amount of fat in the diet. Factors such as late pregnancy and late menopause increase the risk only slightly. The more fat that is consumed, saturated or unsaturated, the greater the chance of developing breast cancer due to an increased secretion of the breast hormone, prolactin, which is tumor promoting. In addition, some of the steroids (cholesterol and bile acids) are converted to estrogens by intestinal bacteria. Estrogens are directly or indirectly responsible for causing cancer.

Dr. Wynder recommends no more than 10 to 20% fat in the diet and no more than 100 mg of cholesterol a day. Americans presently consume more than 40% fat and 600 mg of cholesterol. Women with increased risk due to the presence of non-malignant breast disease should especially follow a diet low in cholesterol and fat.

Overconsumption of fats also affects the production and metabolism of sex hormones in men, often leading to an enlarged prostate gland. The prostate lies just below the bladder and encircles the urethra. It can increase up to ten times its normal size, obstructing the urethra and causing difficulty in urinating. Approximately half the men in America over fifty

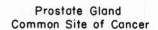

Prostate Gland
Common Site of Cancer

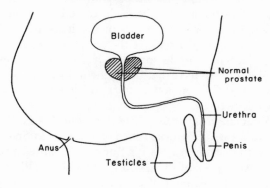

have some degree of enlargement and they are much more likely to develop prostate cancer. South African and Japanese men have a lower risk of developing this kind of cancer until they eat a high-fat diet. The metabolism of sex hormones in American men on a vegetarian diet is more similar to that of South African men eating the traditional diet. Dietary induced imbalance of sex hormones is thought to be the main reason for the increasing incidence of breast, ovary, uterine, and prostate cancer in Western countries.

Osteoporosis: Many adults, especially the elderly, suffer loss of bone tissue although sufficient calcium is found in many foods. When too much fat is consumed, it will combine with calcium in the intestine and form compounds which cannot be absorbed. Another way fat contributes to osteoporosis is by the formation of acid ketones which cause minerals to leave the bones to neutralize the acids. Although our diet may contain ample calcium, excessive fats prevent the efficient absorption and cause it to be leached from the bones. Both of these factors can lead to calcium deficiency and contribute to the development of osteoporosis.

Diabetes: Of the 10 million diabetics in this country 8½ million suffer from the adult onset type. The remaining 1½ million have juvenile onset diabetes, a condition where not enough insulin is secreted into the blood by the beta cells of the pancreas. With adult onset diabetes there is almost never a lack of insulin, especially during the initial stages of the disease. In fact, these people usually have insulin levels that are higher than normal. They are usually overweight, partly because they overeat, but partly because a high level of insulin is a cause of obesity. Their diets are far too high in sugar and fat. Fats cause the insulin to be inefficient in maintaining the blood sugar at normal levels. In an effort to lower the blood sugar, the pancreas puts out more insulin but this does not help.

Many of these people take insulin to control their diabetes, which obviously is not the solution to the problem. If they were to sufficiently decrease the amount of fat they eat, their blood sugar levels would drop to normal in a very short time. Sometimes, however, if they have been on very high doses of insulin for a prolonged period of time, they will have become insulin-dependent. They have become accustomed to receiving insulin from an outside source, and the pancreas stops producing it. In this case, there is nothing they can do but continue taking insulin, since it is absolutely necessary for carbohydrate metabolism. This is called an iatrogenic disease, which means that it is caused by the method of treatment. Fortunately, a test has been devised to determine whether the pancreas is still doing its job. If it is, fats should be severely curtailed in the diet.

Excessive amounts of insulin can lead to arterial disease. If fats are overconsumed they make insulin ineffective. To compensate, the body produces more insulin which stimulates the formation of more fats. This insulin-induced fat formation can cause arterial disease and is one of the reasons most diabetics are overweight.

Diabetes is more common among groups that eat a low-carbohydrate, high-fat diet. The lower the diet in fat the better it is because a low fat diet reduces the insulin requirements of diabetics.

Gallbladder Disease: At the Bowman Gray School of Medicine in North Carolina, squirrel monkeys were used in an experiment which demonstrated that polyunsaturated safflower oil causes more gallbladder stones than do either butter or coconut oil, both of which are highly saturated.

Other factors such as total fat in the diet and the consumption of refined foods contribute to gallbladder disease. (See *Dietary Fiber*.)

Damage to the Enzymes: When excessive amounts of unsaturated oils are consumed, many free radicals are formed causing damage to proteins in the body. Enzymes are composed entirely or partially of protein and when they are altered, it results in a change in the manner in which they react chemically. Sometimes they lose their ability to catalyze the essential chemical reactions in the body. Eventually, the altered chemistry within a cell leads to its death. The loss of function of the cells in an organ contributes to its degeneration.

Immunologic Diseases: Because of mutations caused by the oxidation of lipids, excessive amounts of dietary fats are implicated in the etiology of immunologic diseases including arthritis. It has been suggested that mutated cells stimulate the body's immune system to initiate reactions that tear down the body.

Lipids are substances which the body needs. If excessive amounts are consumed, however, it will result in the development of various degenerative diseases. These include diabetes, atherosclerosis, which is the leading cause of death in the U.S., and many forms of cancer. The consumption of fats and oils is implicated in the etiology of these diseases regardless of their degree of saturation.

The substitution of unsaturated oils for saturated fats may cause more harm than good. This is an extremely important finding and one of which the American public is, for the most part, unfortunately, not aware. It is essential to realize that we must curtail our intake of all fats regardless of the degree of saturation.

Most recipes can be modified by simply omitting any oils or fats. A little imagination and creativity in the kitchen can prolong your life and make it healthier.

Chapter 6

PROTEINS

The body uses proteins in countless ways. More than fifty percent of the dry weight of the cell is protein. It is the principal component of muscle tissue and an important constituent of connective tissue, cartilage and bone. Protein comprises a basic part of our genetic material, skin, hair, mucous secretions, the lubricating fluid in joints, and cell membranes. Proteins play a role in memory and the transmission of nerve impulses.

PHYSIOLOGICAL FUNCTIONS

Osmotic Pressure: Proteins are large molecules, too large to leave the blood stream. Inside the blood they exert osmotic pressure causing fluid to be drawn from between the cells into the blood. This flow of fluid prevents swelling of the tissues and maintains adequate blood volume. Starving people lose protein from all tissues, including the blood. Consequently they often suffer from excess fluids and appear fatter than they really are.

Buffering Action: Proteins can react either as acids or bases. When too much alkali is present in body fluids, proteins act as acids, neutralizing them. In the presence of excess acid, they will act as bases. This way proteins help maintain the body in a slightly alkaline state of pH 7.2. This is critical for normal metabolism to take place.

Hormones: Hormones are protein substances made by cells of various organs or parts of the body and carried to other places where they exert specific effects. Hormones are extremely potent and only exist in minute amounts. They regulate all the body processes including those involved in metabolism. Hormones regulate our growth and the rate at which minerals leave and enter the bones. They control blood pressure, stimulate the formation of red blood cells and produce sex characteristics. Examples of hormones are thyroxine, an iodine-containing hormone regulating growth and metabolism; insulin, controlling the level of sugar in the blood; and adrenaline, that stimulates the breakdown of liver glycogen into glucose. In order to maintain equilibrium, the effects of some hormones are countered by others. For instance, adrenaline acts as an anti-insulin hormone.

Antibodies: Some proteins work to protect us against foreign substances in our bodies, including toxins that cause disease. These protective proteins are called antibodies. Specific antibodies are formed against each toxin we encounter. Sometimes this protective mechanism attacks substances in the food we eat or in the air we breathe. When this happens we experience an allergy.

Clotting: Protein substances cause our blood to clot. In their absence we would bleed to death from minor cuts or injuries.

Transportation: Many substances become attached to proteins in the blood and are thereby transported throughout the body. Fat is rendered soluble in the blood by becoming attached to protein. Fat-soluble vitamins, such as vitamin A, are also transported in this manner. Hemoglobin, a protein in the red blood cells, carries oxygen to the other cells of the body and carbon dioxide from the cells to the lungs.

Enzymes: Enzymes control almost all chemical processes in living organisms. They are catalytic substances, made of protein, that cause organic material to be broken down, changed or assembled. They play a vital role in breaking down our food so it can be assimilated.

Normally, carbohydrates, fats, and proteins could only be metabolized in the presence of strong chemicals or high heat. Enzymes are catalysts: they facilitate chemical reactions so they can take place under milder conditions. Each enzyme catalyzes a different kind of chemical reaction.

Salivary amylase or ptyalin is an enzyme present in the mouth. It initiates the breakdown of starches. Most of the digestion of carbohydrates occurs in the small intestine with the catalytic aid of the enzymes maltase, sucrase, lactase, and pancreatic amylase.

Fats and other lipids are digested in the small intestine by enzymes called lipases secreted by the pancreas and cells in the intestinal wall.

Proteins are digested both in the stomach and in the small intestine by several protein-splitting enzymes called proteases. Without the aid of the proteases, it would take 50 years to digest the protein contained in one meal.

CHEMISTRY

Proteins are large, complex molecules. Like carbohydrates and fats they are comprised of carbon, hydrogen, and oxygen. In addition, however, they contain another very important element—nitrogen—which is needed by all plants and animals. Some of them also contain sulfur. Plants obtain nitrogen from compounds in the soil and they use it to synthesize the proteins they need. Animals, including man, obtain nitrogen by feeding on plants or on animals that eat plants.

As carbohydrates are composed of units of sugar, proteins are made up of building blocks called amino acids. There are twenty-two different amino acids. They are so-called because they contain an amino group and an acid group.

There may be hundreds of amino acids in the protein chain.

The amino acids are connected by peptide linkages. When only two amino acids are joined, it is called a dipeptide. When many amino acids are in the peptide chain it is called a polypeptide.

WHAT HAPPENS TO PROTEIN IN THE BODY

Unlike carbohydrates and fats, protein digestion begins in the stomach where protein is cleaved into smaller pieces called polypeptides. In the duodenum, the first portion of the small intestine, other enzymes break the polypeptides into smaller peptide particles. Eventually the peptides are broken into individual amino acids.

Amino acids are absorbed through the intestinal wall and enter capillaries leading to the portal vein which, in turn, carries them to the liver. Here they are absorbed and formed into huge protein molecules, or packages, in proportion to the usual needs of the various cells of the body. This is an efficient way of meeting the cells' needs.

The packages are released into the blood and carried to the cells, where they are absorbed and broken down into individual amino acids. The cells use the amino acids for protein-synthesis and the excess amino acids are returned to the liver.

Amino Acid / Protein
Absorption and Distribution

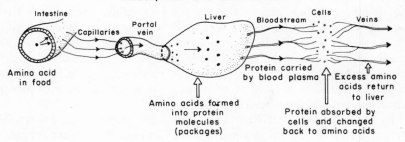

When nutrients combine with oxygen in the cells, by-products are formed. With different fuels there are different by-products. Some of them are easier for the body to eliminate than others. For instance, the by-products of carbohydrate metabolism are easily eliminated through the lungs or the urine. However, the waste products of protein metabolism are not as easily removed from the body. Once the proteins have separated into individual amino acids, the amino group is removed and becomes ammonia. At this point the remainder of the amino acid can be used to form a different amino acid or can be converted to glucose. If excess protein is consumed some amino acids are changed to fat or acetone bodies.

In carbohydrate or fat metabolism, when hydrogen and carbon combine with oxygen to form the waste products water and carbon dioxide, they move to a state of lower energy. The energy released is utilized by the body. However, it is more difficult for the body to rid itself of the waste products of protein breakdown. For nitrogen to combine with oxygen, energy is required, not released. The nitrogen, therefore, remains combined with hydrogen in the form of ammonia, which is extremely toxic to the body. In the liver, a molecule of carbon dioxide combines with two molecules of ammonia to form urea which is excreted in the urine.

Plants must also rid themselves of ammonia and they frequently do so in the form of nitrogen-containing compounds called alkaloids, which exert potent physiological effects. Ergot, strychnine, and the opium alkaloids are examples of these nitrogen compounds. Protein is necessary for the body, but its metabolic products are toxic. We shouldn't eat more than we require.

QUANTITY AND TYPE REQUIRED

Because of its importance, you probably think you need a lot of protein in your diet. This is not the case. Human requirements for this nutrient are relatively small. We should eat only about the amount the body needs each day. It is better to eat enough carbohydrates so we don't have to use protein for energy. Amino acids are used for energy only when the body is not receiving enough calories from other sources.

The Senate Select Committee on Nutrition and Human Needs recommends no more than 12% of the calories we consume each day be from protein. We actually fare better with lesser amounts. In a report issued in 1979, the Federal Trade Commission acknowledged that Americans grossly misunderstand the role of protein in the diet, believing more protein is needed than is the case. The misconceptions regarding protein stem in part from results of early experiments using weanling rats with protein requirements different from our own.

In 1968 the National Research Council set protein requirements between 46 and 56 g. a day, depending on sex and age. The higher amount is equivalent to 2 oz. Since then, the RDA (Recommended Dietary Allowance) has been lowered to 30 to 35 g. daily. In setting this figure, the Council established the minimum amount of protein needed by measuring the amount of nitrogen excreted by 154 lb.-men fed a protein-free diet.

They excreted only 0.8 oz—23.8 g.—which is the amount of protein we need to replace.

The RDA, however, was set higher to account for individual differences. The enlarged amount is higher than necessary and most people could eat much less and still fill their needs. In fact, the body can readily adapt to small quantities of protein by excreting less nitrogen. The oppositeeffect results when large amounts of protein are eaten, the body becomes less efficient in its use of protein.

Most Americans are geting too much protein. Dr. Jean Mayer claims it is virtually impossible in this country to be deficient in protein or any amino acids if you get enough calories and aren't an alcoholic. Only people who are not consuming enough food will be deficient in protein. This occurs occasionally among the elderly. However, even with this group, protein is usually the nutrient in which they are least deficient.

People in underdeveloped countries who do not get enough to eat suffer from what was once identified as protein-deficiency disease. However, they are really suffering from a deficiency of calories. Until the moment of death from starvation, the body converts fats and proteins, either from food or from the body itself, into glucose. Sufficient protein may be provided in the diet, and undernourished people may be lacking only sufficient calories. When a diet is inadequate in protein it will usually be even more inadequate in other nutrients.

As our cells break down, the body puts their protein to use. Each day a half pound of the lining of the walls of the intestine sloughs off. This amounts to 25 to 30 g. (1 oz.) of protein. There are also proteins liberated from the breakdown of enzymes. This amounts to about 150 gms. of protein per day. Protein from discarded cells and secretions contains all the essential amino acids that are found in food.

By a process called transamination, one amino acid can be changed to another. However, animals differ in their ability to make those they need. Man can't synthesize eight amino acids in sufficient amounts and, therefore, they are called the essential amino acids. The requirement for them is small. For adults, only about 15% of ingested nitrogen need come from them. These amino acids are isoleucine, leucine, lycine, methionine, phenylalanine, threonine, tryptophan, and valine. Histidine is also essential for infants.

Complete proteins are those containing the eight essential amino acids in approximately the proportions needed by the human body. Meat contains myosin which resembles the protein in the human body. Therefore, meat is considered a complete protein. Dairy products and eggs are considered by some to contain proteins of even higher quality. According to those who stress the importance of complete proteins in the diet, the protein in eggs is of higher quality than in any other food.

However, proteins are not used by the body in the form in which they are consumed. They are first taken apart into the individual amino acid constituents and then repackaged according to the human body's requirements. If an organism could live on proteins packaged only as they were used, cattle, horses, sheep, goats, etc. could not satisfy their protein needs by eating plants.

Protein is contained in all foods, but in varying amounts and proportions. Some foods are high in certain essential amino acids and low in others. Complementing proteins is the term used when foods that are low in one essential amino acid are combined with foods high in that amino acid. For example, grains are deficient in lysine but high in methionine. Legumes and dairy products are high in lysine. It takes only a very small amount of milk added to cereal to make a complete protein. Some people purposely combine certain foods in order to complement the proteins and provide complete proteins in the diet. However, if your diet is varied and contains sufficient calories, all the essential amino acids will be provided.

The "quality" of proteins is no longer considered as important as it once was. It is almost impossible even for vegans who do not consume eggs or dairy products to eat a diet too low in protein if you get enough calories. Adequate protein will be supplied by a diet of cereals and vegetables and most vegetarians get about three times more protein than they need. The vigorous Tarahumara Indians of Mexico obtain 90% of their calories from corn and beans. However they exceed their requirements for essential amino acids by 236% to 1,121%!

It is impossible to calculate the exact proportions of various amino acids one consumes at a specific meal or on any given day with our present state of knowledge. Requirements for many amino acids depend on the amounts of others present in the body. In fact, studies have demonstrated humans can maintain nitrogen balance when the only amino acids they receive are lysine and threonine. Other essential amino acids are formed by trans-amination.

In developed countries, where caloric needs are easily met, it is virtually impossible for a person to obtain insufficient amounts of any of the amino acids. Although a disease state would result from protein deficiency, no known disease is due to a deficiency of any of the amino acids. The amount of protein, rather than the kind, is the important factor.

MYTHS

Many myths and misinformation exist regarding protein. For many years it was considered advantageous to include large amounts of protein in the diet. In the meantime, research has shown our need for this nutrient is not as great as was once believed.

Athletes and Protein: It is a myth that athletes and people who engage in strenuous activity need more protein than sedentary people. The Tarahumara Indians are an example of superb athletes who consume little protein. Approximately 50,000 Tarahumaras live at a high elevation in the Sierra Madre Mountains of Mexico. They subsist mainly on beans, corn, and squash, and eat little animal protein. They live strenuous lives and often play a form of kickball in which they may run as many as 200 miles.

MINIMUM PROTEIN REQUIREMENT VS.PROTEIN SUPPLIED IN VARIOUS DIETS

	grams protein/day
Minimum Required	35-40
Average American Diet	90-100
Lacto-Ovo Vegetarian	98
Vegan Diet	83

Source: Palombo, J. D. and Blackburn, G. L. Heeman Protein Requirements. *Contemporary Nutrition* 5(1), 1980.

Athletes perspire heavily and lose nitrogen in the sweat. It was believed this necessitated an increase in protein consumption. However, to compensate a smaller amount of nitrogen is lost in the urine.

Enlightened coaches are now meeting the increased caloric needs of athletes by increasing the amount of carbohydrates in their diets. Excess protein can work against the athlete by interfering with water balance. Only during periods of muscle building are small amounts of extra protein needed. This amounts to merely 25 g. (less than 1 oz.) and is met by increased intake of food to meet caloric expenditure.

Protein Diets and Weight Loss: Unfortunately, many people believe a high protein/low carbohydrate diet causes weight loss. However, carbohydrates and proteins contribute the same number of calories—4 per 100 g. The only way to lose weight is to consume fewer calories. Contrary to popular belief, eating protein does not cause body fat to be burned. It has, in fact, been found that high levels of protein can change your metabolism so you actually gain weight.

It is also commonly believed that high protein diets will cause a loss of appetite. Actually, they only cause a loss of appetite for the foods permissible on these diets. It is difficult to get used to eating fats and proteins without carbohydrates. Therefore, fewer calories may be consumed, only because one eats less.

Protein and Fatigue: Another myth holds that increasing the intake of protein reduces fatigue. Energy reduces fatigue and the most efficient sources of energy for the human body are carbohydrate foods.

WHAT TO EAT—WHAT TO AVOID

When people think of protein, they usually visualize a big steak or a hamburger. Meat does not, however, contain as much protein as people think. Most of the calories in meat come from fat, even when all visible fat has been removed. (See *Foods.*)

Eggs, too, are thought of when protein is mentioned. It was once believed the best source of protein was the egg. Rats grew fastest when the protein in their diet came from eggs. However, it has since been found that the protein requirements of young rats are quite different from those of people. Now we realize that 63% of the calories in eggs are from fat. And, a single egg contains more cholesterol than we should obtain each day.

Milk and dairy products should also be limited unless they have been defatted. Almost half of the calories in whole milk are from fat, 30% from sugar and less than one fourth from protein. (See *Foods.*)

Nuts are thought to be a good source of protein. However, they too are a rich source of fat. For example 9% of the calories from English walnuts are derived from protein, but a whopping 88% are from fat. For protein we should rely on whole grains, legumes, skim milk, potatoes, and other vegetables. We require less than 10% of our calories from protein. Wheat contains 20%; beans, 26%; skim milk, 40%; potatoes, 11%; mushrooms, 39%; and lettuce, 29%.

It isn't necessary to worry about sufficient protein when you substitute grain for meat. Meat is very high in fat which contains more than twice as many calories per gram as carbohydrate. Grains and legumes contain less protein than equal amounts of meat, but consuming larger quantities will provide sufficient protein without all the extra fat.

PROBLEMS OF PROTEIN OVERCONSUMPTION

Hypernatremic Dehydration: Waste products of carbohydrate and fat metabolism are easily excreted from the body. Urea, the waste product of protein metabolism, however, requires fairly large amounts of water for its elimination. This is especially true in infants whose kidneys have not matured enough to concentrate the urine very well. The infant will have a higher proportion of water relative to waste products. Protein accounts for only about 6% of the calories contained in human milk. If even small amounts of protein supplements are given to an infant without increasing his water intake, the concentration of urea will increase. This causes more water to be excreted. The result may be a state of hypernatremic dehydration, which can cause brain damage, kidney failure, or death.

RELATIVE AMOUNTS OF PROTEIN IN DIFFERENT TYPES OF MILK

	Protein per 100 Grams	Total Calories	Calories From Protein	Percent of Total Calories in Protein
Human Milk	1.1	77	4.4	5.7
Whole Milk	3.5	66	14.0	21.2
Skim Milk	3.6	36	14.4	40.0

Babies should not be fed skim milk. The protein content is high whereas the calories are low (see chart). Thus the infant must drink so much skim milk to meet his caloric need that he consumes more protein than he needs. If skim milk is the only food an infant receives it can lead to hypernatremic dehydration.

Osteoporosis: Osteoporosis is atrophy or shrinking of the bone mass due to resorption of minerals stored in the bone tissue. It occurs in almost all people in Western countries, usually beginning around the age of thirty-five. The rate of resorption increases with age.

Because bones become weakened, there is an increased incidence of fractures. Thigh bone fractures are one of the leading causes of hospitalization of women over seventy. Vertebral compression fractures are also common and sometimes cause chronic back pain, especially if the vertebrae become deformed rapidly. Changes in the vertebrae cause curvature of the spine which is why older people become shorter. Although osteoporosis occurs with frequency among the elderly in industrialized areas, it is not an inevitable consequence of the aging process.

A diet high in protein is one of several factors associated with the development of osteoporosis. Most protein foods, especially meat, contain minerals (mainly phosphorus) that form acids in the body. To neutralize the acids, minerals are drawn from the bones, resulting in elevated levels of calcium in the blood. Excess calcium is eliminated by the kidneys and lost in the urine. Therefore, people who consume large amounts of protein may have too little calcium in their bones even when their dietary intake is high. This phenomenon was demonstrated in a group of men fed low, medium, and high protein diets and given small, moderate, and large amounts of calcium. More calcium was retained by the subjects on the low than on the medium or high protein diets.

Eskimos, whose diet is even higher in protein than ours, show evidence of bone loss at an even earlier age than we do. Loss of bone minerals was found in Eskimos at age 20, whereas it was not evident in Wisconsin women until age 55 and in men until age 65. On the other hand, the bone density of British vegetarians in all age groups was significantly greater than in non-vegetarian control subjects.

Calcium is not the only mineral excreted by the body in increased amounts when protein intake is high. Studies show when more than 90 g. a day of protein are consumed, more phosphorus, zinc, and magnesium are also excreted.

Ketosis: Many dieters adhere to high protein diets including large amounts of meat, dairy products and eggs. They deliberately exclude carbohydrates as too fattening. They hold the mistaken belief that these diets cause permanent weight loss.

In the absence of carbohydrates, dietary fats are converted to ketone bodies. The accumulation of these toxic ketones in the blood is called ketosis and requires large amounts of water for their elimination. The resultant dehydration accounts for weight loss during the first few days of such a diet. On resuming a normal diet, water will be retained and the weight quickly regained.

Ketone bodies compete with other waste products, such as uric acid, for excretion. Excess uric acid can lead to gout, kidney stones, or kidney damage.

Complications with Kidney Disease: Diets high in protein are dangerous for people with kidney damage. Urea and other waste products of protein metabolism are removed from the blood by the kidneys. If the kidneys are diseased, urea can accumulate to toxic levels in the blood. This condition is called uremia and can cause mild symptoms such as loss of energy, appetite, and weight, or it can result in convulsions, coma, and death.

Kidneys also help regulate the acid-base balance by ridding the body of excess phosphates and sulfates, most of which come from protein. If too much protein is eaten by someone with kidney damage, electrolyte imbalance may result making it impossible for the body to maintain its optimum acid-base balance.

Complications with Liver Damage: High protein diets can be dangerous for a person with liver disease. During the digestion of protein, bacteria in the intestine produce the waste, ammonia, which is carried by the portal vein to the liver. Additional ammonia is produced during the metabolism of protein in the liver cells. Since even small amounts of ammonia are extremely toxic to the central nervous system, especially the brain, it is quickly converted by the liver to urea which is less toxic and easily excreted. In the presence of liver damage less ammonia is converted to urea, and it enters the blood instead. Unless people with liver disease restrict protein, they will develop protein intoxication. This involves a malfunctioning of the brain and can lead to coma or death. In fact, sensitivity to protein is sometimes the first sign of liver damage.

Atherosclerosis: Hypoxia is the term used to describe subnormal levels of oxygen in the blood. Some researchers think hypoxia, which can be caused by increased amounts of protein in the blood, is a significant factor in the development of atherosclerosis. High protein diets also contribute to atherosclerosis because they include large amounts of animal food and therefore are high in fat and cholesterol.

Cancer: The incidence of cancer is higher among meat-eaters than among vegetarians. This was thought to be due to the larger amount of fat in the diet of meat-eaters. Recent studies indicate the fat in meat may not be the only culprit. It has been found that rats fed higher amounts of protein developed more cancer than those fed lower amounts. It is hypothesized that animal products might cause a modification of the bacteria growing in the intestine. More research is needed in this area.

Large amounts of protein are definitely *not* good for us. We obtain some protein from almost every food and it is not necessary to eat highly concentrated protein foods. Because protein increases the rate of growth, it was once thought that large amounts were integral to a good diet. High protein diets make cattle bigger and fatter more quickly, but the purpose of human nutrition is to ensure a long, healthy life.

Chapter 7

DIETARY FIBER

Dietary fiber is that portion of plant foods *not* broken down by our digestive enzymes. It is the structural material of plants and is found mainly in their cell walls.

Fiber is not a single entity but a complex of carbohydrate and non-carbohydrate components such as celluloses, hemicelluloses, pectins, gums, mucilages, and lignin. Each component of the fiber complex has different physical and chemical properties. Fiber is not a good name for this complex since not all of these constituents are fibrous. Dietary fiber used to be referred to as roughage. This term is also inaccurate since fiber absorbs water in the digestive tract making the feces soft—not rough.

There are billions of bacteria in the large intestine. They break down some of the dietary fiber but only a small amount is absorbed by the body. Its energy contribution is insignificant; humans derive only 5% of the potential energy contained in fiber. Therefore, when fiber is removed from foods in processing, the result is food that is more highly concentrated in available calories.

Although fiber contributes very few calories to our diet, it is not an inert substance. It performs invaluable biological functions. It gives bulk to the feces, facilitating the transit of fecal material through the intestine. It inhibits the formation of toxic matter in the intestines and prevents the absorption of many substances. It also dilutes the concentration of substances in the intestine that would damage it. It serves to dilute the calories of food making overconsumption less likely. And, it discourages the growth of harmful bacteria.

SOURCES OF FIBER

Most fiber in the American diet comes from wheat. However, all grains contain large amounts before they are refined. Legumes are another rich source, while vegetables and fruit contain more water and less fiber. In general, the cell walls of fruit (especially summer fruit) are thin and contain less fiber. Apples and citrus, although containing relatively small amounts of total fiber, are high in a fiber constituent called pectin which is especially effective in reducing cholesterol in the blood. Nuts and seeds are high in fiber, but should be eaten in small quantities because they are also high in fat.

If necessary, a diet can be supplemented with unprocessed bran. It is better, however, to rely on a varied diet of whole, unrefined foods to supply the fiber we need. There are many benefits from eating foods containing all the natural constituents of fiber, while the addition of individual fiber components will not give the same effects. For instance, cellulose is sometimes added to commercial high-fiber breads. While it serves to dilute the calories, it doesn't afford other benefits of naturally occurring fiber such as protection against excessive clot formation. Unrefined carbohydrate foods contain all the different forms of fiber.

Don't rely on food tables and charts to calculate the amount of fiber in foods. Most tables show the amount of crude fiber rather than dietary fiber. Crude fiber is that which does not break down when fiber is extracted in the laboratory with strong chemical solvents. Dietary fiber, on the other hand, is that which is not broken down in our bodies. Since conditions in our body are milder, the amount of dietary fiber in our food is substantially greater than the amount of crude fiber. For instance, whole wheat flour is 2% crude fiber and 11% dietary fiber.

Man has adapted to a diet high in fiber. The size of primates correlates with the type of diet eaten. Small primates eat food containing less fiber; their diets are concentrated in calories. The smaller they are, the higher their diet is in insects, fruits, and sap. The structure of the cells of their intestinal tracts allows them to use such concentrated foods.

The diet of larger primates is different. Among the great apes, which are similar to man, the larger the animal the more fiber in the diet. Leaves comprise more than 90% of the diet of a 400 lb. gorilla and only about 25% of the diet of a 100 lb. chimpanzee.

In developing countries, 75% of the diet is in the form of starchy foods. In this century, the diet of Western countries has undergone radical changes. Inhabitants of the industrialized countries adhere to a diet where only 30% of the calories derive from starchy foods. Not only does the diet contain a much smaller percentage of these foods, but almost all of the fiber has been removed. The transition from the traditional diet to that of today has resulted in fiber intake decreasing from 24 to 6 g. a day. The removal of fiber from our food has led to many health problems.

Different kinds of plant foods contain different proportions of fiber constituents and you must include many types of fiber foods in the diet to receive the full benefits. Some people, notably the elderly, may not consume enough food to provide adequate amounts of fiber. Often when people lose their teeth they experience difficulty in chewing and delete grains from their diet. Supplements of unprocessed bran will help with constipation problems. Small amounts of bran can be added to the diet daily, with gradual increases. The bran should be mixed with food or liquid to prevent the chance of inhaling it.

EFFECTS OF UNDERCONSUMPTION OF FIBER

Constipation: The most obvious problem associated with a lack of fiber is constipation. We are a constipated nation, spending huge sums of money on laxatives. Approximately a quarter of all elderly people who visit physicians complain of constipation.

Fiber retains large amounts of water in the intestines giving bulk to the fecal mass and allowing it to move more rapidly through the colon. Insufficient fiber in the diet causes contents of the digestive tract to move more slowly, leaving time for much of the water to be absorbed. This causes the feces to become hard and small, diminishing the stimulus to defecate. Hence small feces are retained for a longer time.

A diet high in fiber also helps to combat constipation in another way. It is believed some of the waste products from bacterial digestion of fiber in the intestines can have a cathartic effect. In other words, when the bacteria degrade certain kinds of fiber, substances are produced that irritate the intestines causing them to propel the contents at a faster rate.

People from underdeveloped areas who migrate to industrialized countries become constipated when they forsake their traditional diet. This is a complaint of many African and Indian students in the United Kingdom. It does not take long for them to become as constipated as the British. Even rabbits fed a diet of white bread, butter, milk, sugar and vitamins become fat and constipated.

The following chart will illustrate the difference in stool weight and transit time of food through the gastrointestinal tract among people in Africa, India, and Western countries.

STOOL WEIGHT AND TRANSIT TIME

Africa and India	300-500 g.	30-35 hr.
Western countries	100 g.	3 days – 2 wks.

Adding fiber to the diet will not cause diarrhea. Fiber normalizes bowel function. Since it retains water it prevents both hard and loose stools. Some foods are more effective than others in relieving constipation by increasing stool weight. It takes only about 2 oz. of whole wheat bread a day to double your stool weight. In comparison, you would have to eat 3 times as much white bread, 4½ times as much carrots, 5½ times as much cabbage, and 18 times as much apples.

Hemorrhoids: Half the people over fifty in North America suffer from hemorrhoids. Hemorrhoids are varicosities or dilations of the delicate hemorrhoidal veins in the anus. They are extremely vulnerable to the presence of hard feces and straining during defecation. The mass of dilated veins results in swelling about the size of your small fingernail. As the swellings increase in size, they can be pushed through the anus when defecating. Because they are irritated whenever the bowels are moved, they are apt to become inflamed.

The result is pain, itching, and sometimes bleeding. Once hemorrhoids have developed, fiber is recommended to soften the stool and prevent further irritation of the damaged vessels. Avoiding constipation usually prevents hemorrhoids.

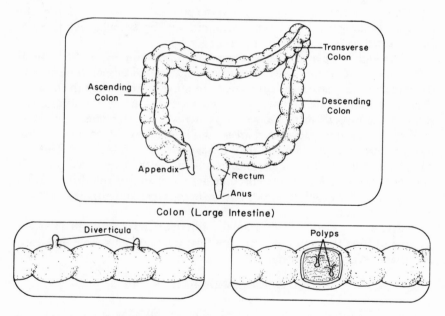

Colon (Large Intestine)

Diverticular Disease: The colon is divided into sections. When the muscles that encircle the back part of a section contract, that portion is closed and the lower part opens. The longitudinal muscles then contract, propelling the fecal mass forward. This task is easily accomplished when there is sufficient fiber in the diet and the contents of the colon are large and soft. However, small, hard feces cause the muscles to work harder. The resulting increase in pressure can cause a ballooning out of the colon wall. Little pockets, diverticula, are formed. The sigmoid colon exerts the most intense contractions and is, therefore, the site of most diverticula. The condition is called diverticulosis.

Food particles can become lodged in the diverticula causing inflammation. The hard feces pass more slowly through the colon allowing the multiplication of bacteria. The stretched and irritated walls of the diverticula become infected. This is called diverticulitis. Diverticular disease is the most common of all intestinal diseases in North America. It afflicts 30% of those over 60 years of age.

Two British researchers, Denis Burkitt and Hugh Trowell, have engaged in valuable research on dietary fiber and its effect in the prevention of diverticular disease. They noted there has been a dramatic increase in the disease in the past seventy years. Dr. Burkitt is a surgeon who spent twenty years at a teaching hospital in Uganda. He found a total absence of diverticular disease in rural Africa. These researchers feel the remarkable differences in the health of American and African intestines can be explained by the absence of fiber in the American diet.

During war, industrialized countries see a significant decline in the number of deaths due to degenerative diseases. This has been attributed to the scarcity of sugar, fat and meat. Atherosclerosis and other degenerative diseases decreased dramatically in Britain during the First World War. However, the incidence of diverticulosis remained the same because the British were still able to obtain refined grains.

The incidence of diverticular disease in Japan is increasing as their diet becomes similar to ours. In India and Iran, diverticulosis is seen only in the upper classes; they alone consume a diet low in residue. Diverticulosis can even be induced in rats and rabbits by removing fiber from the diet. Until recently, a low fiber diet was prescribed for the treatment of diverticulosis. Now there has been a reversal in this thinking and most physicians recommend adding fiber to the diet of their patients. Fiber might not cure diverticulosis, but it controls it. However, some foods such as seeds, nuts, and berries may still have to be avoided because they are too irritating.

Ulcerative Colitis: Dr. Trowell implicates low fiber diets in the causation of ulcerative colitis. This disease is characterized by inflammation of the colon and the presence of bleeding sores exuding purulent matter, fibrin, and mucus. The patient suffers with cramps and diarrhea. It is usually a chronic disease, with intermittent attacks, and a danger of sudden hemorrhaging or rupture.

Ulcerative colitis is rare in undeveloped countries. Jews in the Middle East do not have this condition until they move to Israel where a large part of their diet consists of refined foods. In our country, it is more common in urban than rural areas, in the North than in the South, in private than in county hospitals, and among the educated than the uneducated. It used to occur with only a third the frequency among U.S. blacks but it is increasing. In France, where more vegetables are eaten, there is a lower incidence of ulcerative colitis than in other developed countries.

Treatment of ulcerative colitis should be left to the physician. However, it can be *prevented* by the consumption of high fiber, starchy foods.

Spastic or Irritable Colon: This condition is characterized by abdominal pain, alternation between constipation and diarrhea, and the passing of mucus and very small stools. The abdominal pain is a result of violent contractions of the lower colon. The condition is misnamed; instead of irritable colon, it should be called *irritated* colon. It is caused by the same diet that causes diverticular disease and is thought to be its precursor. If left untreated, the condition can degenerate into ulcerative colitis and increase the risk of developing bowel cancer. After an attack of colitis has subsided, treatment is an increase of fiber in the diet. Excessive amounts of raw fruits and vegetables, however, should be avoided.

Spastic colon is found even among young people and is often the result of sloppy eating habits. Teenagers and young adults too often satisfy their hunger quickly with energy-rich, low fiber foods. Although emotional turmoil can exacerbate the condition, it is not thought to be a factor in causing spastic colon.

Colorectal Cancer: People with a low intake of fiber have a greater risk of developing colorectal cancer. The colon accounts for about five feet of the large intestine and the rectum is the terminal five inches. This kind of cancer accounts for more deaths in the United States than any other.

The colon contains hundreds of types of bacteria. Some are harmless, but others, such as the bifidobacteria, are equipped with enzymes that can break down bile acids into powerful cancer-causing substances. The intestinal contents remain in the body for a longer period in people on a low fiber diet. This slow passage time allows the bacteria to convert more of the bile acids into carcinogens. It has been demonstrated in rats that a high fiber diet protects against chemically induced bowel cancer.

The bacterial flora in the gut can be changed by diet. A high fiber diet tends to cause a predominance of the so-called "friendly bacteria." Low fiber diets cause a predominance of the bacteria that degrade bile acids into carcinogens. Fiber also dilutes any carcinogenic substances that might be present, so fewer intestinal cells come in contact with them.

Malignant and benign polyps (tumors) occur in the same people and are thought to be due to the same cause. Most polyps don't become malignant but most cancer of the large bowel develops from these polyps. Small polyps are seen in almost 70% of autopsy examinations in Western countries. However, over a twelve year period, polyps were seen in only six of 14,000 autopsies in a hospital in Africa.

The incidence of colorectal cancer is related to the wealth of a population more than any other disease. In the United States, colon cancer used to be much more common than in the rest of the world. Now, however, the discrepancy is lessening as other people become more affluent.

Appendicitis: Appendicitis is an inflammation of the vermiform appendix. This organ is a sac-like appendage protruding from the cecum at the juncture of the small and large intestines. Hard pieces of fecal matter—fecoliths—are found in the appendices of patients undergoing appendectomies. Fecoliths obstruct the appendix, causing it to become swollen. Intestinal contents become trapped inside, bacteria propagate, and the appendix becomes infected. Fecoliths are not formed in the soft feces of people on high fiber diets.

The cause of appendicitis was recognized 60 years ago. It was rare until the end of the nineteenth century; since then it has become common in most civilized countries paralleling a change to a low fiber diet. As with diverticulitis, the First World War saw no decrease in appendicitis in Britain because refined flour was still available. Appendicitis was ten times more common among wealthy boys in an English boarding school than in a large orphanage where coarse food was served.

Rural Africa has a very small incidence of appendicitis, although it is seen more frequently in the urbanized areas. Japanese living in Hawaii experience more appendicitis than those in Japan because their diet includes more refined foods. On the other hand, Dutch POW's in Japan during World War II experienced a decrease in appendicitis because their diet consisted mainly of coarse vegetables.

Varicose Veins and Phlebitis: Varicosities of the veins are due to increased abdominal pressure caused by straining to relieve the bowels when constipated. This pressure is transmitted down the veins of the legs causing dilation or varicosity. Sometimes the veins become inflamed resulting in phlebitis, which is often painful.

It was once thought varicose veins were caused by prolonged standing. However, it has been shown the condition is only aggravated by standing, not caused by it. Varicosities of the leg veins often appear, or worsen, during pregnancy because expectant mothers in Western countries often suffer from constipation. If the diet contains adequate fiber a woman can bear many children with no varicosities.

Pulmonary Embolism: Our veins contain valves to prevent the backward flow of blood. With continued pressure from straining during constipation, the valves eventually become ineffectual allowing the blood to flow back down the veins. The slow moving blood allows the formation of clots which become attached to the already damaged vein wall. If a clot becomes detached it is called an embolus. Emboli from the legs usually find their way through the blood system to the arteries in the lungs. Here they cause obstruction—pulmonary embolism. The part of the lung supplied by the blocked artery loses its function; pulmonary embolism is a leading cause of death. A diet high in fiber helps prevent this condition.

There is another way in which fiber helps protect against the formation of clots. Fibrinolysis, a process by which blood clots are dissolved, is decreased when we eat a diet high in fats and low in fiber. Clots in African Bantus dissolve twice as fast as they do in Europeans, and the rate doesn't decrease with age. Fibrinolysis in rural Bantus, however, occurs at a faster rate than in urban Bantus.

Peptic Ulcers: Peptic ulcers are sores caused by digestive juices. They can occur in the lower portion of the stomach. Usually, however, they are found in the upper portion of the duodenum, the first part of the intestine.

Although the mechanism by which fiber-containing foods protects against ulcers is not clear, they are rare in undeveloped countries and common in countries eating a highly refined diet. Studies in India and Africa indicate there is no clear correlation between smoking, caffeine, alcohol, or the consumption of spices and the development of ulcers. These may worsen the condition but they do not cause it.

Almost no ulcers were seen among American troops during the First World War, but they were a major cause of disability during World War II. Studies of the effect of diet on prisoners during the Second World War shed light on the origin of ulcers. American prisoners in Singapore were given both milled rice and the polishings—the nutritious part of the grain removed during milling. However, in 1943, the polishings were no longer available, and by 1944 there was a high incidence of ulcers. In Hong Kong, prisoners were fed milled rice. The incidence of ulcers—many of them perforated—was high. After two years, many of these prisoners were transferred to Japan where they were fed unmilled rice. Their ulcers disappeared.

Ulcers were very common among soldiers in the German army. It was found, however, that the troops closest to the front lines had fewer cases. They were subjected to much greater stress but the food they ate was crude. There were also very few ulcers among German prisoners in Russia due to their diet of cabbage and unrefined grains.

Diabetes: In poor societies, large amounts of complex carbohydrates are eaten. When these people become wealthier they begin to consume more sugar and the incidence of diabetes increases proportionately.

The inhabitants of the island of Nauru in the Pacific have become wealthy from exporting phosphate. They lead a leisurely life and import refined food. Thirty percent of the islanders over the age of 15 have diabetes.

When South African Bantus and New Zealand Maoris moved into towns, they began to replace fiber-containing foods with large amounts of sugar and the incidence of diabetes increased. This was also seen among the Yemenite Jews who migrated to Israel. In the Yemen, little sugar is eaten and diabetes is practically unknown. When they migrate to Israel, the amount of sugar in the diet increases greatly, and among those who have been there for twenty years, there is a huge increase in the incidence of the disease.

In our own country, there are 10 million diabetics. The greatest incidence is seen among the Pima Indians in Arizona. They eat a large amount of refined foods and are generally obese. Testing indicates that 50% of the Pimas over 35 are diabetic.

In Britain, flour containing 72% of the wheat berry was formerly used in bread making. In 1941 the government raised it to 86% of the wheat berry. Between 1941 and 1953, the rate of death due to diabetes dropped 54%. The commercial bread flour in the United States still contains only 72% of the wheat berry.

Insulin is more efficient in lowering blood sugar levels when the diet includes fiber. Just how fiber improves glucose tolerance is not clearly understood. One theory holds that gel-forming constituents of fiber cause the intestinal contents to be less liquid. Therefore sugar and other nutrients are absorbed at a slower, more even rate. The most advanced and effective treatment of diabetes is a diet low in fat and sugar, and high in complex carbohydrates. This type of therapy is also without the harmful side effects of drug treatment.

Tooth Decay: Tooth decay and disease of the gums is also associated with a refined diet. According to Dr. Abdul Adatia, from the University of Bristol Dental School, refined starches are the most cariogenic food. Cavities are not common among people living in unindustrialized environments.

In 1932, 83% of the people who lived on Tristan da Cunha, an island in the South Atlantic, were free of tooth decay. They ate fish, potatoes, milk, eggs, and green vegetables. In 1942, a store was established and refined foods became readily available to the islanders. Ten years later, only 22% of the population was cavity free.

Unrefined foods, according to Dr. Adatia, contain factors such as phytates which cause tooth enamel to be more resistant to decay. Chewing causes these substances to be released, and fiber in foods necessitates more chewing.

Gallbladder Disease: Some researchers are convinced that a refined diet lacking in fiber is also responsible for stones formed in the gallbladder. The liver manufactures bile, a fluid containing cholesterol and bile salts which are made from cholesterol. Bile is secreted by the liver into the gallbladder, a hollow pear-shaped organ lying under the liver. The bile becomes concentrated and is stored here until food enters the intestine; then it is discharged into the intestine. Its function is to emulsify fats, making it easier for them to be digested. Almost all bile salts are reabsorbed at the end of the small intestine and are returned to and recycled by the liver.

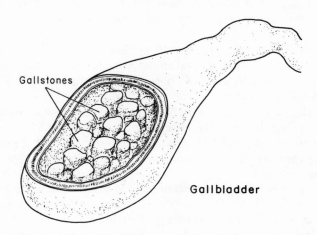

Gallstones

Gallbladder

When adequate fiber is consumed, bile salts bind to it, are carried through the large bowel and are excreted in the feces. The liver must then dip into the body's supply of cholesterol to produce more bile acids. This is the main way the body rids itself of cholesterol.

When excessive amounts of calories are consumed, the cholesterol in the bile becomes concentrated. Refined foods cause the liver to produce fewer bile salts. These salts act as emulsifiers keeping the cholesterol in the bile in solution. When the amount of cholesterol increases and the bile salts decrease, the bile becomes supersaturated and cholesterol crystals precipitate out. These crystals act as nuclei around which the stones or calculi form.

If a stone becomes lodged in the tube leading from the gallbladder to the duodenum, it results in inflammation of the gallbladder. The severe contractions of the gallbladder trying to empty itself results in excruciating pain. Gallbladder disease is common in all Western countries. It is especially common among American Indians, especially the Pimas; 73% of Pima women have gallstones.

The incidence of gallbladder disease has increased at an astonishing rate since the Second World War. Since then, there has been a corresponding decrease in the consumption of whole grains accompanied by an increase in the consumption of sugar. Whereas gallbladder disease used to be seen among the middle-aged and the elderly, it now affects even younger people in Western countries.

Atherosclerosis: Fiber binds bile acids causing them to be excreted, thereby calling on the body's supply of cholesterol to replace them. Therefore people on high fiber diets have lower levels of cholesterol and triglycerides in the blood and are at lower risk of developing atherosclerosis.

Eleven hundred pairs of brothers who grew up in Ireland were studied. When grown, one of each pair moved to Massachusetts, and they were compared with the remaining brother for evidence of heart disease. It was found that 4% of those who had migrated had diseased coronary arteries, while only 2.1% in Ireland did. The Irish brothers ate more potatoes, bread, and whole grain cereals—foods rich in natural fiber.

Many Jews from Middle Eastern countries migrate to Israel where the diet is highly refined. Before emigrating, their serum cholesterol levels were low but quickly increased when their diets changed.

Hiatus Hernia: Hiatus hernia is another disorder we suspect is caused by lack of fiber in the diet. The esophagus passes through an opening in the diaphragm, called the esophageal hiatus, and then empties into the stomach. Hiatus hernia refers to a condition where part of the stomach protrudes up into the chest cavity. This area of the stomach no longer functions properly and gastric juices back up resulting in pain and occasional bleeding.

Hiatus hernia is one of the most common defects of the gastrointestinal tract in developed countries and is rare in less developed countries. Based on epidemiologic evidence, it is associated with a lack of fiber in the diet. It is caused by straining due to constipation. Straining increases the intra-abdominal pressure and pushes part of the stomach up through the diaphragm.

The removal of fiber from our food has been one of the most drastic changes in the diet of Western man. Dr. Denis Burkitt says that in Britain and the United States so much fiber has been taken out of our food we pass small stools and need large hospitals. Because of the alarming rate of increase in medical costs, it would behoove us to increase the size of our stools.

Chapter 8

VITAMINS

Vitamins are organic substances essential to the healthy functioning of our bodies. They are needed in small amounts and either can't be produced by our bodies at all, or in amounts adequate to the maintenance of optimum health. Individual vitamins usually function as parts of enzymes with which they combine. They enable the body's enzymes to use the food we eat and perform important chemical reactions in the body.

Nutrition is a relatively new field and the study of vitamins is in its infancy. Until the second decade of the twentieth century vitamins were not even known. At first they were called "vitamines." The root of this word derives from the fact these substances are vital to the functioning of the body. The suffix, "amines," refers to nitrogen-containing substances. In 1920 the "e" was dropped when it was discovered that most vitamins don't contain nitrogen. Although we have learned much about these small nutrients in a short time, the total effect of a given vitamin is still not generally understood. Vitamins are often taken to cure an isolated symptom, while we remain unaware of other effects they may have on us. Nor do we understand the complex interrelationships between vitamins and other nutrients.

Vitamins fall into two classifications—water-soluble and fat-soluble. Water-soluble vitamins include vitamin C and members of the B-complex. Fat-soluble vitamins include vitamins A, D, E, and K. It is a myth that only fat-soluble vitamins can cause toxicity. It was thought water-soluble vitamins would be washed out of the body in urine if an overdose was taken. Although fat-soluble vitamins are stored longer in the body, increasing the risk of accumulation to toxic levels, some water-soluble vitamins are capable of being stored for a relatively long period too.

Acute vitamin deficiency will lead to disease. Deficiency diseases are seen frequently in times of famine and in underdeveloped countries that cannot produce sufficient food to meet the needs of their populations. These diseases are rarely experienced in industrialized countries and most physicians in America have seen them only in textbooks.

115

Symptoms of minimal vitamin deficiency in Western countries are usually caused by eating too much of the wrong kind of food—food from which the nutritional ingredients have been removed by processing. Also, eating too much of the wrong kind of food can cause an increased demand for certain vitamins. The deficiencies in this country usually do not result in clinically evident disease. Instead we have such symptoms as insomnia, headache, loss of appetite, nervousness, or a general rundown feeling.

The amount of vitamins we need can only be discussed in general terms. Not only do individual needs vary, but many complex interactions exist between various vitamins themselves and the food we eat. This is an area where much is still to be learned. Our needs for various nutrients, including vitamins, vary with our diet, environment, age, emotions, heredity, and physical health.

The best way to ensure enough vitamins is to eat a well-balanced diet of unrefined, whole foods. Keep in mind that vitamins are packaged in a balanced manner by nature, and you are unlikely to get an excess or deficiency of any single vitamin if you eat a variety of whole foods. When taking vitamins in the form of foods exactly as they are found in nature, there is little chance of misuse.

Extracted vitamins, "vitamin pills," are drugs just like any other substance extracted from plant or animal materials or produced synthetically for therapeutic purposes. Although vitamins are generally less toxic than other drugs they can be abused. Some people think if a little is good, more is better. Such a philosophy can be especially dangerous when mothers overdose their infants with vitamins and minerals. A small dose for an adult can be an overdose for an infant. In addition, babies have yet to develop the mechanisms in their bodies that would detoxify drugs, making them more susceptible to any kind of poisoning. Until the exact biochemical functions of vitamins are known, and until we understand the interrelationships among them, it is far better to eat a balanced diet than to rely on vitamin pills.

RDAS

The *Ninth Edition of Recommended Dietary Allowances* (RDAs) was published in 1980 by a Special Committee on Dietary Allowances appointed by the Food and Nutrition Board of the National Academy of Sciences. The RDAs were first established in 1943 as a guide to help plan the nutrition of the armed forces during the Second World War. RDAs are based on studies determining the amount of a nutrient that must be ingested if intake is to equal the amount lost from the body each day.

The RDAs are set at levels high enough to meet the needs of most people. For example, when the required amount of a nutrient is determined, it is often doubled to establish the RDA. Most people, therefore, require less of the nutrients than the amounts recommended. There is continuing controversy over the RDAs and they are revised every four or five years.

The RDAs should not be confused with the minimum daily requirements (MDRs) which were established many years ago by the Food and Drug Administration as a standard for labelling in the food industry. They have never been revised and are out-of-date.

Vitamins have been measured in international units (IU), milligrams and micrograms. In the past, the fat-soluble vitamins—A, D, and E—were calculated in international units. However, this has been discontinued, and now all nutrient recommendations are given in terms of weight. Vitamins A and D are listed in micrograms (mcg.) and vitamin E in milligrams (mg.).

1 gram (g) = 1000 milligrams (mg) = 1,000,000 micrograms (mcg)

MEGAVITAMIN THERAPY

The optimum vitamin requirements of most people can be met with good diet. It is best to maintain health through controlling the quality of the diet. There are, however, a few people whose vitamin requirements will not be satisfied by any diet. In this case it is best to find a physician who is trained in metabolic disorders and is familiar with vitamin therapy.

Vitamins are not foods—they are parts of foods. When used in their extracted form, rather than as parts of whole foods, they are being used as drugs. The symptoms and side effects of overdose should be listed on the label.

In recent years some physicians have claimed success treating mentally ill patients, especially schizophrenics, with megavitamin therapy. Thousands of times the normal requirements of certain B vitamins have been used in these treatments. Some psychiatrists refute these claims, and further studies haven't corroborated the theory. We need more research to determine whether certain mental illnesses are, in fact, metabolic disorders. It will be interesting to see the results of future studies in this area.

COMMON SOURCES OF VITAMINS

Vitamin	Destroyed By	Sources
Thiamin	Use of baking soda or excessive temperature, time or heat in cooking	Practically all plant and animal tissues —whole grains—meat, especially pork —dairy products—fruits—vegetables
Riboflavin	Sunlight	Whole grains—fruits—nuts—leafy vegetables—fish meat—dairy products, especially milk—eggs

Niacin	Excessive water in cooking (fairly stable)	Meat—fish—whole wheat—peas —broccoli—potatoes—tomatoes
Vitamin B_6	Extreme heat in processing	Whole grains—legumes—bananas —potatoes—cabbage—meat—in all animal and plant tissues to some extent
Pantothenic acid	Dry heat, acidity or alkalinity	Almost all foods
Biotin	Avidin (in raw egg whites)	Milk—whole grains—legumes—nuts —eggs—meat, especially chicken
Folacin	Prolonged cooking or storage	Vegetables, especially leafy—fruits—meats —eggs
Vitamin B_{12}	Stable	Dairy products (lesser amounts in yogurt than in non-fermented dairy products)— meat—eggs—miso— soy sauce
Vitamin C	Heat—light—air (Very unstable)	All fresh fruits and vegetables, especially citrus, peppers, green vegetables
Vitamin A (active form)	Oxidation during processing (fairly stable)	Butterfat (higher in summer than in winter)—liver
Vitamin A (carotene)	Oxidation during processing (fairly stable)	Yellow and green vegetables, especially carrots, sweet potatoes, squash, papaya and leafy vegetables
Vitamin D (active form)	Stable	Made by the body when skin exposed to sunlight—fish liver oil
Vitamin E	Heat—Light —Air	All oil-containing foods— lettuce and other green vegetables—whole grains —legumes
Vitamin K	Oxidation—Light	Meat—leafy vegetables —alfalfa —milk—liver—eggs—Endogenous source: intestinal bacteria
Vitamin F	Oxidation	All foods of plant origin

B VITAMINS

The B vitamins are water soluble. With the exception of B_{12} they occur together in the same foods. They work together activating enzymes that influence the chemical reactions involved in the breakdown of food into energy. The system does not work unless all are present. They also assist in synthesizing sugars, amino acids, and fats.

Thiamin: In 1880, one-third of the Imperial Japanese Navy died of a disease later named beriberi. First the sailors became weak and lost weight, then they became paralyzed as degenerative changes in the nervous system occurred. It was first thought the disease was caused by an infective organism, but none was found. The sailors' diet consisted of a little fish and seaweed and much polished rice. British sailors, however, weren't afflicted by this insidious disease. For a while it was thought the rice contained a harmful substance but this idea was rejected because the peasants at home ate rice and they didn't get sick.

The sailors were eating a fine rice imported from the British and French colonies. It took a long time to realize that it was not something in this rice that was killing the Japanese sailors, but they were dying because something had been *removed*. The polished rice lacked thiamin. This is now the preferred term for what was first called vitamin B_1, the first B vitamin discovered.

Thiamin is a necessary part of an enzyme essential in the breakdown of carbohydrates. In thiamin deficiency, certain breakdown products of carbohydrate metabolism will accumulate in the blood to toxic levels. These toxins are responsible for the symptoms of beriberi. Symptoms of mild deficiency include loss of appetite, fatigue, and constipation. These symptoms can be due to a variety of causes.

Thiamin supplements can interfere with the processes of normal metabolism. Too much thiamin causes a deficiency of pyridoxine, another B vitamin. Excess amounts of this vitamin can cause shingles, hyperthyroidism, allergic-like reactions, and even anaphylactic shock—a type of shock caused by an allergen in sensitive people. Extreme reactions to thiamin, however, are rare.

Riboflavin: Riboflavin is a bright yellow powder; when added to water it has a yellow-green fluorescence. It is necessary for the activation of enzymes essential in the metabolism of carbohydrates. One of these enzymes catalyzes several important chemical reactions.

Riboflavin is easily destroyed by light. Maybe you remember the old-fashioned brown glass milk bottles. They prevented the destruction of the riboflavin when milk was left by the milkman on your front porch. Opaque milk cartons today accomplish the same purpose.

Symptoms of riboflavin deficiency include cheilosis (lesions in the corners of the mouth), eye lesions, and excessive capillary growth in the cornea. It is very difficult to know which of the B vitamins is causing a particular symptom. Lesions can result from thiamin, riboflavin or niacin deficiency and are difficult to distinguish. Since you may not know which deficiency you may have, it can be dangerous to take vitamins without undergoing tests to determine your vitamin nutriture. If you take a vitamin in which you are not deficient, it can create a greater deficiency of one in which you really are deficient.

Niacin: Niacin is also known as nicotinic acid or vitamin B_3. More than forty chemical reactions in our bodies are dependent on this vitamin.

A severe deficiency of niacin causes pellagra. The word is derived from the Italian *"pelle agra,"* rough skin, which becomes pigmented like a blotchy sun tan and then rough and scaly. There is inflammation of the mucous membranes of the mouth, tongue, stomach and intestines. The afflicted stagger at first; then their legs become paralyzed. Paralysis spreads to other parts of the body, and the disease eventually leads to death. Some of the dying have black tongues, and some experience terrifying hallucinations.

Pellagra occurs among the poor or during times of famine when corn is the basis of the diet. During the Napoleonic Wars, European farmers were forced to sell their livestock and vegetables and subsisted almost entirely on corn. Pellagra became epidemic and it was realized that this dreadful disease was associated with corn. As with beriberi, it was thought either the corn had spoiled or was infected with a dangerous organism. Needless to say, the consumption of corn in Europe was reduced drastically, and since that time, Europeans have used it almost exclusively as animal fodder.

In the United States, however, corn continues to be a staple in many areas. In 1913 many cases of pellagra appeared in the rural South. It was finally realized that people who lived almost exclusively on corn were not getting enough of a newly discovered vitamin—niacin. Corn contains all the B vitamins, but the niacin is bound very tightly to other substances and is not released in the body.

Indians in Mexico and Peru have eaten huge quantities of corn since ancient times without developing pellagra. They were protected because they ate beans along with their tortillas. Since corn was not the only food in their diet, they obtained niacin from another source. They also treated the corn with lime, which makes the niacin more available and also adds greatly to the calcium content.

If you take niacin, watch for symptoms of overdose. Flushing, headache, cramps, and nausea can be caused by taking only 300 mg. of niacin. Larger doses can cause itching and pigmentation of the skin. Gram doses can cause liver damage.

Vitamin B_6: Although frequently called pyridoxine, B_6 is a group of three vitamins—pyridoxine, pyridoxal, and pyridoxamine. It is necessary for the activation of the enzyme that converts the glycogen (carbohydrate stored in the liver) to glucose, and aids in the metabolism of protein.

Symptoms of deficiency are loss of appetite, weight loss, and weakness. However, B_6 deficiency is rarely seen since our diet usually provides all we need. It was once seen in infants whose only source of nourishment was a commercial formula that had been heated so much in processing that vitamin B_6 was destroyed. No toxic side effects have been observed.

Pantothenic Acid: Pan means "all" in Greek and this vitamin was so named because it exists in all unrefined foods. Like other B vitamins it is essential to the metabolism of the food we eat. We obtain at least two to three times the amount of this vitamin we require in our normal diet. Deficiency was observed in malnourished prisoners of war suffering from vascular disease that resulted in malalgia or the "Burning Feet" syndrome. No toxicity has been seen even when large doses of this vitamin were taken.

Biotin: Biotin is produced by bacteria in the intestine and is easily absorbed from that site. In order to produce deficiency in humans, it was necessary to feed volunteers a diet containing a large number of raw egg whites a day. Egg white contains a protein substance called avidin which is an anti-vitamin. It combines with the biotin in the intestine, preventing its absorption. Biotin deficiency seen in the volunteers manifested itself in dermatitis, depression, fatigue and muscle pain.

In experimental animals fed a purified diet, this vitamin prevented greying and loss of hair. PABA, folic acid, and inositol also prevented hair greying in animals. They have not been found to have the same effect in humans, however.

Folacin: This vitamin gets its name from foliaceous or leafy vegetables. Folacin is converted to an acid, which is vital for the multiplication of cells and is necessary for red blood cells to develop from immature cells into normally functioning adult cells.

Although folacin is abundant in foods, it can be destroyed by overcooking or prolonged and improper storage. Deficiency is sometimes seen among elderly people who do not include leafy vegetables in their diet. It is also seen in malnourished pregnant women who have a greater need for this nutrient.

Deficiency of folacin causes megaloblastic anemia, and was often seen in pregnant women in India in the 1930s. In this type of anemia there are too few normal and too many immature red blood cells—megaloblasts. Women who take oral contraceptives have an increased need for this vitamin, too.

Folacin cannot be purchased in amounts larger than 0.1 mg. without a prescription from a physician. This is because treatment with folacin masks some symptoms of pernicious anemia, a dangerous deficiency caused by lack of vitamin B_{12}. To make sure you get enough of this vitamin, include a large salad in your daily diet. And remember, prolonged cooking destroys folacin.

Vitamin B_{12}: is unlike the other B vitamins because it can be synthesized only by bacteria. Our intestines house bacteria that produce this vitamin, but they are too low in the intestine for us to absorb it. We must obtain B_{12} by ingesting the bacteria that produce it, by eating animals who have ingested these bacteria, or by eating animal products such as milk and eggs. Products such as soy sauce or miso which are fermented by bacteria are also sources of B_{12}. Yeasts do not synthesize B_{12}. However, they are often grown on cultures containing B_{12} and some is absorbed.

Vitamin B_{12} deficiency leads to a rare disease, pernicious anemia. Symptoms include weakness, sore tongue, numbness and tingling of the extremities, loss of appetite, pallor, diarrhea, difficulty in breathing, rapid and sometimes irregular pulse, dizziness, ringing in the ears, pain in the upper abdomen, and heart failure. Loss of coordination of the lower extremities and fingers results from damage to the spinal cord and peripheral nerves. If untreated, damage to the nervous system may result in paralysis.

In 1926 it was discovered that eating a half pound of *raw* liver a day cured symptoms of the disease. With the discovery of vitamin B_{12} in 1948, it was realized that pernicious anemia was a vitamin deficiency disease. In order to absorb this large vitamin, a certain protein substance must be present in the gastric juice. People with pernicious anemia are unable to produce this substance or there is an impairment of its activity. They can absorb B_{12} in sufficient amounts only if they eat raw liver daily. Now, however, intramuscular vitamin shots are the prescribed treatment. Fortunately, the daily need for B_{12} is low and it is readily stored in the liver. Therefore large and infrequent doses can be administered to these patients.

Vitamin B_{12} is a lovely red colored liquid. This seems to make it very desirable for its placebo effect. It has been used to treat patients who complain of fatigue although the symptom is completely unrelated to the need for the vitamin. Sometimes it is requested by athletes who attribute magical powers to the red substance. Because excess amounts are easily excreted, it is not harmful.

Vegetarians who include eggs or dairy products in the diet do not need B_{12} supplements. To be on the safe side, strict vegetarians who consume neither animal nor bacterial-fermented products should take an occasional supplement. These supplements can be obtained from non-animal sources. For vegetarians who consume dairy products, a daily half glass of milk, skim or whole, will provide ample B_{12} in the diet.

If you are not a strict vegetarian you are getting ample B_{12}. This vitamin is not damaged by ordinary cooking although it can be destroyed by the extreme temperatures used in processing. For example, 90% of it can be lost in making evaporated milk. The body conserves B_{12} efficiently and when none is ingested it usually takes decades for deficiency to become manifest.

Choline, Inositol, PABA, Amygdalin (Laetrile), Pangamic Acid, and Orotic Acid: Some people think these substances are B vitamins. Choline, inositol, and PABA are essential for normal metabolism and are found in the same foods as the B vitamins. They are, however, not considered vitamins by most nutritionists. Amygdalin has been called vitamin B_{17}, pangamic acid has been marketed as vitamin B_{15}, and orotic acid has been labeled B_{13}.

Choline is made in the body but may need to be supplemented by dietary sources. When it was excluded from the diet of some experimental animals, they experienced a fatty infiltration of the liver as well as hemorrhagic kidney disease. Choline is part of lecithin which acts as an emulsifier of fats in the intestine.

Inositol is a sugar-like substance with a sweet taste. It is synthesized by all plants and animals. It has been claimed by those who advocate supplementation that inositol protects against atherosclerosis. Research has not borne this out. It has, in fact, been found to cause slightly elevated levels of cholesterol and other lipids in the blood. No specific need for inositol or symptoms of deficiency have been found, although it is assumed to have an important function.

PABA is necessary for normal coloration of rat fur. For this reason, the popular press recommended it to prevent greyness in humans, although subsequent research found no validity in this claim. PABA is found in all plant and animal tissues and is synthesized by humans. It is used as a sunblocking element in suntan lotions.

Amygdalin (Laetrile), pangamic acid and orotic acid have all been called "vitamins," usually by those who want to promote their usage. There is no evidence, however, that they are essential to human metabolism. Amygdalin, also called Laetrile, is found in the pits of such fruits as almonds, apricots, cherries, plums, etc. and has been called vitamin B_{17}. Laetrile, derived from apricot pits, is claimed as a cancer cure. This is highly controversial and should be studied further. Opponents of Laetrile usage claim this treatment is dangerous and is often used as a substitute for therapy that might be more effective.

Pangamic acid, sometimes called calcium pangamate, has been marketed under the name "vitamin B_{15}." It can be obtained in some health food stores and there are claims that it will cure a wide variety of ailments. There is no standard of identity for pangamic acid and it contains varying amounts of substances with different properties. Some of these substances are inert but others have adverse effects, especially the chloride substances. These are toxic and strongly suspected of being mutagenic and carcinogenic. The sale of these products is illegal and they have been seized by the Food and Drug Administration many times. The sale of "vitamin B_{15}" has been prohibited in Canada for more than ten years.

Another exotic sounding substance, orotic acid, has been called "vitamin B_{13}." There are claims that a deficiency of orotic acid may lead to premature aging. This claim will guarantee large sales when it becomes available.

VITAMIN C (ASCORBIC ACID)

Since ancient times sailors were afflicted with scurvy. Initially their gums would bleed, become sore and inflamed. They would lose their teeth, become weak, and their legs would swell. Death would be caused by scurvy or secondary infections. It was thought scurvy was caused by an infective organism. An English ship once put a man in the final stages of the disease ashore on an island so the other members of the crew would not catch the disease. He was so weak he could only lie where he was placed. To satisfy his hunger, he plucked at the grass around him and ate it. Gradually he felt stronger and began eating fruits and berries growing on the island. He made a speedy recovery and was eventually rescued. The sailor was cured because the grass and other vegetation on the island contained what later came to be known as vitamin C. On shipboard, the usual fare was salted fish, smoked meat, bread and hardtack. None of these foods contained vitamin C, which is found in all fresh fruits and vegetables.

The fact that the abandoned sailor recuperated after eating a little grass demonstrates how small a quantity of this vitamin is required to prevent scurvy. The officers on board ship stayed healthy because they ate a somewhat more varied diet. Even an occasional potato prevented the disease.

British sailors used to be referred to as limeys because they realized this relatively non-perishable fruit would prevent scurvy. However, some sailors who drank lime juice still got sick, because they boiled it. Vitamin C is easily destroyed by heat, air, and light. Processed foods or foods stored for long periods of time lose much of their vitamin C content. Frozen vegetables lose about 50% and frozen fruit about 30%.

Vitamin C is a sugar-like substance. Most animals possess an enzyme which enables them to synthesize sufficient amounts of the vitamin from glucose. However, this enzyme is lacking in man, monkeys, guinea pigs, the Indian fruit bat, and the red-vented bulbul bird. Some people may be able to synthesize small amounts of vitamin C, but not enough for health. Vitamin C is necessary for the adrenal glands to synthesize adrenaline and anti-inflammatory steroids. It is also needed for the formation of connective tissue that holds cells together; therefore it is necessary for tissue repair. It may also stimulate the immune system. Illness or other kinds of physical stress such as smoking or adverse environmental conditions encountered in polluted cities, increases our need for this vitamin.

The daily requirement for vitamin C is easily met by a half a cantaloupe, a grapefruit, an orange, a cup and a half of coleslaw, or a large baked potato. It is found in all fresh fruits and vegetables and it would be difficult to become deficient unless these foods were completely omitted from the diet. This too often occurs with the elderly.

The use of megadoses of vitamin C has become controversial. Vitamin C is thought to stimulate the immune system when consumed at the recommended levels. However, if taken in excessive amounts, it may have a negative effect. In 1970 Linus Pauling published the book, *Vitamin C and the Common Cold*, wherein he advocated huge doses of vitamin C to combat colds, measles, mumps, chicken pox, pneumonia, hepatitis, the flu, and cancer, and to increase longevity. A Canadian researcher set out to disprove Dr. Pauling's theories regarding vitamin C and the common cold. The results of this reliable study were quite different from those expected. The group given vitamin C experienced fewer sick days than those given the placebo. Other researchers have been unable to duplicate these results. Whether this is due to lower doses or for other reasons is not clear.

Dr. Pauling also studied the effect of vitamin C on terminal cancer patients. Those who took the vitamin lived an average of four times longer than those who did not—200 days compared with 50 days. This study should have been followed up by studies on a larger scale. The National Cancer Institute has finally decided to do further testing of vitamin C on terminal cancer patients. Such studies are also being carried on in other countries. It will be fascinating to see the results.

There are arguments against large doses of vitamin C. Prolonged usage can cause dependency. When excessive amounts are taken, mechanisms for its destruction become activated. If a person suddenly stops taking the large doses, a temporary deficiency could result. A corollary problem can occur in babies. When pregnant women take more vitamin C than they need, their babies are born with a dependency on larger amounts. When this dependency isn't met, infantile scurvy develops. Infantile scurvy has been seen in babies born to mothers who took 400 mg. of vitamin C a day during pregnancy.

Some studies have found that the weak antihistaminic action of vitamin C can reduce the severity of the symptoms of a cold, but it can cause the cold to last longer. Excessive amounts of vitamin C have also been implicated as a cause of kidney stones. Ascorbic acid is partly metabolized to oxalic acid. Some people form more oxalic acid than others, and they would be at a greater risk of developing stones.

Large doses of vitamin C have also been reported to destroy the vitamin B_{12} we consume. Taking gram quantities of vitamin C can induce vitamin B_{12} deficiency in people whose intake of B_{12} is low. Excessive amounts cause diarrhea. Large doses have also been reported to contribute to urinary stones, hypoglycemia, and abortion in some laboratory animals. The vitamin can also cause damage to the mucous lining of the cervix. Large doses of the vitamin have been found to contribute to the development of atherosclerosis by causing an imbalance in the zinc/copper ratio in the body.

Even if large doses of vitamin C prove beneficial in the treatment and control of infectious diseases or cancer, it does not mean that healthy people should take supplements. An aspirin cures a headache, but the headache was not caused by an aspirin deficiency and it would not be wise to take aspirin on a daily basis to prevent headaches. If vitamin C helps combat cancer, it does not necessarily follow that the cancer was caused by a deficiency of the vitamin or that we should consume it in megadose quantities to prevent it.

It is better to get vitamin C from fruits and vegetables than from pills because foods that contain vitamin C also contain bioflavonoids, substances that protect this very unstable vitamin from oxidation. Vitamin C supplements with bioflavonoids are available but they are more expensive. Other factors that enhance our health may be in complete foods but not found in vitamin tablets. Some people think it is beneficial to take rose hip tablets to get their vitamin C. Actually, rose hips contain very little of the vitamin and the supplements are fortified with synthetic ascorbic acid.

VITAMIN A

During World War I, the Danes could not eat the butter they produced but were forced to sell it and eat margarine. Because butter was their main source of vitamin A, the substitution resulted in an epidemic of a disease of the cornea—xerophthalmia—in Danish children.

Vitamin A is a complex of chemically related substances found only in animal sources such as butterfat, liver, egg yolks, and fish oils. The one exception is spinach which contains small quantities. Vitamin A acts like a hormone but since it can't be made in the body it is classified as a vitamin.

Plant foods do not contain vitamin A but they do contain carotenoids which are precursors of the vitamin. Our bodies readily convert the carotenoids to vitamin A. The carotenoids are yellow and account for the color of carrots, sweet potatoes, cantaloupes and many other fruits and vegetables. Generally, the darker orange or green a vegetable, the higher the carotenoid content. One of the carotenoids, beta-carotene, can be produced synthetically and is used commercially as a safe coloring agent in foods. Vitamin A deficiency could have been prevented in the Danish children if they had been given carotenoid-containing vegetables. Vegetables, however, are not always obtainable in the winter months in northern countries, especially in wartime.

Many thousands of children lose their sight every year due to xerophthalmia. In years of famine as many as a quarter of a million go blind in India, Southeast Asia and parts of Africa and South America. Their sight could be saved if they had only an ounce or two of greens, carrots, or papaya each day. Of course, famines lead to deficiencies in all nutrients but those who survive will never regain their sight, even if they never go hungry again.

The functions of vitamin A are not completely understood but it is known that it helps prevent night blindness; stimulates bone growth; promotes fertility; and is needed for normal formation and health of the inner and outer skin. The inner skin is the mucous membrane lining the intestines and the respiratory passages. Vitamin A is necessary for maintaining the proper amounts of mucous secretions by the cells of the inner skin, and to prevent the cells of the outer skin from becoming rough and dry—keratinized.

It is impossible to accumulate toxic amounts of vitamin A by consuming vegetables rich in carotenoids. Only a certain amount will be converted to vitamin A; the rest will be stored in the skin. Some people consume enormous amounts of carrot juice, turning their skin yellow. This can be unsightly, but it is not injurious.

It is possible, but not likely, to consume toxic amounts of vitamin A from animal sources. Toxicity can be caused by vitamin supplements and the amount that capsules can contain is regulated. Excessive amounts of vitamin A cause loss of appetite, crankiness, blurred vision, dry and irritated skin, hair loss, fatigue, diarrhea and nausea, insomnia, painful bones and joints, abnormal bone growth, and enlargement of the liver. Vitamin A toxicity is more likely to occur in children than in adults. Less than twice the recommended adult dose can cause toxicity in a young child. Large amounts of the vitamin can cause both demineralization of bony tissue and excessive mineralization of the periosteum, the membrane covering the bone. In infants there is a swelling of the soft spot. It is unwise to give supplements of any kind to children unless they have been prescribed. When sub-toxic levels of vitamin A were added to the diets of laboratory animals, cholesterol was deposited in large amounts in the arteries and other tissues.

Several recent studies have investigated the relationship of cancer and vitamin A and chemically related synthetic substances. These studies demonstrated that when experimental animals are deficient in vitamin A, they get cancer of epithelial cells more frequently when exposed to carcinogens. The moral of these studies seems to be a carrot a day might help keep certain kinds of cancer away. The studies should not be interpreted to mean the more vitamin A you take, the less likely you will be to get cancer. It means that adequate amounts will help protect you from this one kind of cancer.

Fat-soluble vitamins are not as easily destroyed as are those that are water-soluble. Prolonged cooking at excessively high temperatures will destroy vitamin A. Carotene, on the other hand, is made more available when vegetables are lightly cooked, pureed or mashed. These processes cause the breakdown of cell walls making the carotene more available.

VITAMIN D

In northern Europe, it was once common to see deformed children among the urban poor who lived in dark slums. They had pathetically thin and grotesquely bowed legs, knock-knees, and their skulls and chests were misshapen. These children were afflicted with rachitis—now called rickets. It is due to a deficiency of vitamin D.

Vitamin D is really a hormone, and is required in minute amounts. Unlike true vitamins, it can be made in the body if the skin is exposed to sunlight. There is a precursor in the skin, which when exposed to ultraviolet light is converted to the active form of the vitamin. Only a small area of the skin (a few inches in diameter) need be exposed to sunlight for a few minutes a day in order for the body to produce adequate amounts. It is not necessary to get out in the sun every day since the vitamin is readily stored in the body.

Vitamin D occurs in large amounts in fish liver oils, and is also found in mackerel, tuna, herring, and salmon. However, sunlight is a much more important source.

Vitamin D facilitates the absorption and use of calcium and phosphorus necessary for normal bone mineralization. In deficiency, the bones become soft. If the condition is not corrected by the time an infant is walking, the result will be skeletal deformities. In children the condition is called rickets. In adults it is called osteomalacia. This often results in back pain and spontaneous fractures. In older people, the condition is usually a result of a malabsorption problem.

It is especially important for young children to receive enough of this vitamin while their bones are growing rapidly. In polluted industrialized areas, the sun's rays are blocked, particularly in northern climates during the long, dark winter months. You can imagine the plight of undernourished black children living in these areas during the time soft coal was burned for heat. Both children and adults deprived of exposure to the sun's rays need to receive vitamin D from dietary sources. This is especially true for dark-skinned people who immigrate to northern countries. The pigmentation in their skins protects them from the harmful effects of overexposure but also prevents them from producing vitamin D as readily as light-skinned people.

Milk, both whole and skim, is fortified with synthetic vitamin D. For this reason, deficiency is no longer the problem it once was. However, the synthetic form of the vitamin is not as effective as that found naturally in food or in the skin, and it is more toxic. Except for elderly shut-ins, adults get enough from diet and normal outdoor activity. Housebound people cannot produce sufficient quantities of vitamin D because ultraviolet rays can't penetrate glass windows. There are special fluorescent bulbs (Vita-Lite) available that produce rays stimulating vitamin D synthesis in the skin. Eight hours of exposure to this kind of lighting is equivalent to a fifteen minute walk at noon in the summer.

It does not require much above the recommended dose of vitamin D to produce symptoms of toxicity. Excessive amounts cause calcium deposits in soft tissues including the lungs, blood vessels and kidneys. Damage to the kidneys can be permanent. It also causes loss of appetite, thirst and irritability. Very small amounts of this vitamin (remember it is a powerful hormone) have potent pharmaceutical effects. An infant should never receive more than 10 micrograms (400 IU). Infants fed cod-liver oil in addition to vitamin D fortified milk and cereals can get too much. Vitamin supplements should never be given to an infant without consulting a physician.

VITAMIN E

This vitamin is a complex of fat-soluble substances called tocopherols. The most active is alpha tocopherol. Other tocopherols are beta, delta, epsilon, eta, gamma and zeta. When they exist together, they are referred to as mixed tocopherols. Foods containing oils such as whole grains, seeds, and nuts are the highest in tocopherols. They are also contained in significant amounts in leafy greens and fish.

Vitamin E combines easily with oxygen thereby preventing oxidation of other substances in the body. Oxidation occurs when a car rusts or food becomes rancid. Vitamin E protects substances in the body from oxidation, including hormones, vitamin A, and the fatty acids, especially those that are unsaturated. Protecting the fatty acids from oxidation helps control the formation of substances that damage and age the cells.

Topical application of vitamin E is an effective treatment in the prevention of excessive scar tissue. However, it does not accelerate the healing process. On the contrary, whereas vitamin A stimulates repair and the synthesis of collagen (the substance that holds cells together), vitamin E has an inhibitory effect.

Some people take vitamin E supplements in the mistaken belief it will improve sexual performance. The belief originated when researchers discovered that rats completely deprived of vitamin E for prolonged periods of time had reproductive problems. It is unlikely any human diet could contain so little of the vitamin that these problems would result. People hearing of these early experiments, however, confused sterility with libido. Vitamin E has no effect on libido or virility.

Vitamin E has been found to be of no use in the treatment or prevention of heart disease. It does not improve circulation but enables more efficient use of oxygen in the blood. Therefore, it has been useful in relieving symptoms of impaired circulation in the legs. Because it functions as an antioxidant, adequate amounts of vitamin E serve to protect against lung damage caused by components of air pollution. Sometimes vitamin E is added to poultry feed to preserve the freshness of meat and to prevent formation of carcinogenic substances.

Deficiency is apt to be the result of a diet composed largely of refined foods and a good deal of vegetable oils. Refined grains—white flour and products made from it—are almost lacking in vitamin E, while extracted vegetable oils create a greater demand for the vitamin. The more oils one consumes, the higher the requirement for vitamin E.

Unlike vitamins A and D, vitamin E supplementation seldom causes acute toxicity in humans although it does in animals. However, supplements of 15 micrograms (600 IU) a day have been found to raise the amount of blood triglycerides in women. Muscular weakness and fatigue have been seen in people taking 10-20 micrograms a day for a week. And, vitamin E creams can cause rashes. Larger amounts interfere with normal thyroid function and can result in increased amounts of cholesterol in the blood.

VITAMIN K

Vitamin K is a group of compounds that have an antihemorrhagic effect. It was discovered in 1934 by a Dane who called it the coagulation vitamin—*Koagulation* in Danish, hence the K. This vitamin is necessary for the formation of blood clots. If the body were unable to form clots we would bleed to death from minor wounds.

Vitamin K is not truly a vitamin as it is synthesized by bacteria in the intestine and easily absorbed. It is also found in many foods such as lean meat, vegetables and milk, and to a lesser extent in fruits and potatoes.

Deficiency occurs only as a result of certain medical problems involving malabsorption or when taking certain drugs such as anticoagulants, aspirin, or some antibiotics. The antibiotics—such as sulfa drugs and the tetracyclines—suppress the growth of bacteria that synthesize the vitamin.

VITAMIN F

Three unsaturated fatty acids—linoleic, linolenic and arachidonic—used to be referred to as vitamin F. Arachidonic is no longer considered an essential fatty acid because it can be synthesized in the body from linoleic acid. Some researchers maintain that it is only necessary to obtain linoleic acid in the diet, but others feel that linolenic is essential, too. These fatty acids play a role in lipid metabolism and the maintenance of cell membranes. They are richly supplied in all oil-containing vegetable foods, especially whole grains, legumes, seeds, and nuts. They are also in such vegetable foods as lettuce. Deficiency is not seen in healthy people eating normal diets, but has been observed in hospital patients receiving intravenous feeding for a long time. Deficiency could also occur in people with a serious disease preventing them from absorbing fats. In this case, the deficiency would not be alleviated by any amount of fatty acids in the diet.

NATURAL VERSUS SYNTHETIC VITAMINS

The relative value of synthetic and natural vitamins is controversial. People in the health food industry claim only natural vitamins—those extracted from foods—are beneficial. Others claim synthetics are identical. So little research has been conducted in this area, it is difficult to broach the subject with much authority. However, because this question is raised so often, I want to tell you what we do know.

Natural and synthetic vitamins are not always the same. Some synthetic vitamins are isomers of vitamins occurring in foods. That means the molecules contain the same elements, but are positioned differently in the molecule. This is also true of amino acids in natural foods compared to synthetic amino acids. They behave differently in the body and synthetic amino acids are harder to digest. Many different sugars are isomers of each other and also have different characteristics.

Synthetic vitamin E is made from turpentine or petroleum and is an isomer of the natural vitamin. Natural vitamin E is processed from tocopherols derived from vegetable oils—usually soybean oil. It reacts differently in the body than the synthetic.

Natural and the commercial synthetic form of vitamin C, however, are exactly the same. Synthetic vitamins are cheaper than natural vitamins, but sometimes contain artificial food coloring. It is usually best to obtain your vitamins from a healthful diet.

DRUGS AND VITAMINS

Drugs do not always mix well with vitamins. They can prevent absorption and utilization of many vitamins and lead to certain deficiencies. Some will prevent the synthesis of vitamins in the body. Mineral oil, sometimes used as a laxative, will prevent the absorption of two fat-soluble vitamins—A and D. Oral contraceptives may increase the need for several nutrients especially folacin and vitamin B_6. Many drugs, including aspirin and barbiturates, increase the requirements for vitamin C. Prolonged use of most antacids depletes the body of thiamin. The antacid, aluminum hydroxide, interferes with the absorption of vitamin D. Diuretics cause the body to lose water-soluble vitamins. Anticonvulsants inhibit the absorption of folacin and vitamin B_{12}. Sugar and alcohol, both of which could technically be considered drugs, cause the body to be depleted of B vitamins. Sometimes vitamin E lowers the insulin requirement of diabetics. And, detoxification of drugs in the body may cause an increased need for certain nutrients.

Barbituates are frequently prescribed for elderly people to help them sleep. Since many older people don't eat balanced diets, they tend to suffer from marginal nutritional deficiencies. In addition, most older people suffer from osteoporosis—the softening and shrinking of bone tissue. Barbiturates will make less calcium available for bone maintenance because they adversely affect metabolism of the vitamin D necessary for the absorption and utilization of calcium. Phenobarbitol has also been found to increase the rate at which vitamin C is excreted from the body. The glucocorticoids, anti-inflammatory drugs used in the treatment of arthritis, have similar effects.

These are just a few of the drugs that interfere with vitamin nutriture. If long-term drug treatment is prescribed for you, ask your doctor about the nutritional implications of such therapy. If necessary, do some research on your own about the drugs you are taking and get him copies of the studies so he can evaluate them. Many drugs are prescribed by specialists who may not know as much about nutrition as an internist or general practitioner. Discuss the drugs you are taking with your family doctor so he can advise you on the proper nutritional regime to accompany your drug therapy.

If you have been taking drugs for a long time, I would recommend Daphne Roe's book, *Drug Induced Nutritional Deficiencies*, Avi Publishing Company, Westbrook, Connecticut. This book will be very helpful when you discuss drug therapy with your doctor. It should not, however, be used as a manual for self-medication with vitamins. I do not recommend self-medication for anyone, especially for those people who are ill enough to be under the care of a physician.

Other forms of medical intervention besides drug therapy can influence the need for many nutrients. Nutrition should be considered before and after surgical procedures and radiotherapy. It is your responsibility to discuss with your physician how you can improve the speed of your recovery through proper diet or with vitamin supplementation. Remember vitamins will deteriorate with age. When they do, they can have adverse effects on the body.

If you take vitamin supplements, stop doing so at least a week before having blood tests. Supplements can cause false results on some tests thereby making diagnosis of your condition more difficult for your doctor. When you go for a medical examination, tell your doctor exactly what supplements you are taking and in what quantities.

Chapter 9

MINERALS

Elements are the basic constituents of our physical world. Some elements, or their ions (individual atoms of an element that have lost one or more electrons or have extra ones in their outer shells), are found in the food we eat—in animal and plant tissues, and in their fluids—and are referred to in nutrition as minerals. After our foods have been broken down in our bodies the minerals remain and are called ash. This ash constitutes about 4% of the body. The rest is composed of carbohydrates, lipids, proteins, and water.

The ash in the body is not inert, but serves extremely important functions. It helps regulate the body's water balance; serves as a component of hormones, enzymes, vitamins, bone, teeth, hair, nails, and intra- and extra-cellular fluids; helps regulate the acid-base balance, maintaining the body at a very slightly alkaline pH; and aids in the function of nerves and muscles.

The various minerals constituting ash must be maintained in the body in delicate balance. Some pathological conditions, extreme diets, or toxicity can overwhelm the mechanisms that maintain the minerals in proper proportions. Healthy people, however, will be able to keep the minerals in proper ratio to each other if a wide variety of unrefined foods is eaten.

Minerals are part of our food and should be obtained from food. When they are ingested in their extracted form (in pills) they are used as drugs and can have potent pharmacological effects. We probably have not yet discovered all the nutrients necessary for optimum health. Consequently we should eat a wide variety of unrefined fresh foods. Minerals are lost during the extreme procedures of food processing. They are not destroyed by heat, light or air but can be leached out in the cooking water. Fruits and vegetables should be eaten raw, steamed or boiled in as little water as possible. The cooking water can be re-used as a tea or soup stock. Food like rice should be cooked in only as much water as it will absorb.

SOURCES OF MINERALS

Minerals	Source
Calcium	Dairy products Leafy vegetables Broccoli Oranges Whole grains Legumes Sweet potatoes Green beans Seafood (especially with bones)
Phosphorus	Animal protein Whole grains Nuts Legumes Carbonated beverages
Magnesium	Whole grains Legumes Dairy products Potatoes Green vegetables
Potassium	All fruit (especially oranges and bananas) Vegetables Potatoes Whole grains Legumes

Sodium	Processed foods (especially cheeses,
	sauerkraut,
	  pickles, olives, potato chips,
	  salted nuts, luncheon
	  meats, etc.)
	Foods of animal origin

Chloride	Meat, including fish and poultry Eggs Grains
Sulfur	Meat Fish Eggs Legumes Cabbage
Iron	Meat, fish & poultry Legumes (especially lima beans)

Whole grains
Leafy greens
Fruit (especially apricots,
  peaches, pears, grapes, and
  plums)
Eggs
Blackstrap molasses
Nuts
Potatoes

Zinc

Meat
Poultry
Fish (especially tuna)
Legumes
Whole grains
Leafy greens (especially
  Brussels sprouts)
Eggs
Milk
Mushrooms

Copper

Whole grains
Legumes
Nuts

Selenium

Fish
Whole grains
Broccoli
Tuna
Garlic
Mushrooms
Radishes
Cabbages
Onions
Carrots
Meat
Milk

Iodide

Deep ocean fish
Plant foods and milk from
  areas where soil contains
  sufficient iodide
Iodized salt

Manganese

Whole grains
Legumes
Foods of plant origin
  (especially leafy greens)
Nuts
Pineapples

Chromium

Whole grains
Meat
Poultry
Milk

Cobalt	Fruit
	Leafy greens
	Milk
	Poultry
Fluoride	Fish
	Water
	Tea
	Small amounts from plant and animal foods
Molybdenum	Whole grains
	Legumes
	Milk
	Dark green vegetables
Silicon	Foods of plant origin

THE SOIL

There are extremists who say our soil is so depleted we cannot obtain enough nutrients from foods grown in it and we must resort to taking large quantities of numerous supplements. Others say the nature of the soil has no bearing on the nutrient content of foods because if the soil does not contain the nutrients needed by plants, they will not grow. There is some truth and a lot of irresponsible exaggeration in both of these claims.

Plants do reflect the type of soil in which they are grown, and have been used as indicators of the amount of minerals in different soils. The amount of minerals in plants, however, is dependent not only on the amount in the soil in which they are grown, but also on such factors as soil acidity and weather conditions.

Vegetation does not thrive in soils deficient in the minerals they require, but plants will grow in soils that provide inadequate amounts of a few minerals required by humans but not by plants. For example, people in the Goiter Belt developed iodide deficiencies because the soil in which their food was grown was deficient. Iodide is not essential to plants, neither are selenium, cobalt or zinc. Such minerals are not involved in the metabolic processes of plants, and their concentration in plant tissues varies widely depending on soil conditions. However, people in sophisticated societies do not consume food grown in only one area. Therefore we are not as affected by local soil conditions as are peoples in more primitive societies. Primitive people satisfy their nutritional requirements with fewer foods. In industrialized countries, we obtain enough of the various minerals by eating from a wide selection of foods.

Some vegetables contain higher amounts of one or more minerals and lesser amounts of others. For instance, lettuce contains generous quantities of iron, iodide, copper, zinc, and calcium, but not much selenium. Cucumbers, on the other hand, contain substantial quantities of selenium but not much of the other minerals. If we eat many kinds of vegetables we will be supplied with ample amounts of all minerals.

MACRONUTRIENT MINERALS

Seven minerals are needed by the body in relatively large amounts, 100 mg./day or more. They are referred to as macronutrient minerals and include calcium, phosphorus, magnesium, potassium, sodium, chloride, and sulfur.

Calcium: Calcium accounts for 2% of our weight; it is the most frequently occurring mineral in the body. As adults our bodies contain two to three pounds of calcium. Almost all the calcium in the body is in the bones and teeth, but a small amount is in the softer tissues—muscle and body fluids. In these tissues, calcium has many important roles to play. In fact, the bones serve as a storage depot for the calcium when it is not needed elsewhere. Approximately 700 mg. of calcium leave and enter the bones each day. The other tissues have priority over the bones, when they need the calcium it leaves the bones and can cause them to become soft and porous. Therefore, if calcium is inadequate, it is the structural tissues that suffer.

Calcium plays a role in the formation of blood clots. If we did not have the ability to form clots we would be in constant danger of uncontrolled bleeding. Clotting is a complicated process and calcium in the blood is one of many factors necessary for it to occur.

Calcium aids the absorption of the large and cumbersome vitamin B_{12} molecule. Since that vitamin is necessary for the health of the nerves, calcium plays an indirect role in the normal functioning of the nervous system. It also plays a more direct role by aiding in the transmission of electrical impulses from one nerve cell to the next. For this reason, calcium is also necessary for the contraction of muscles, including the heart. To maintain a regular heart beat, calcium must be present in the fluid between the heart's cells.

Because nerves and muscles require the presence of calcium in body fluids, many people think it beneficial to take bone meal, dolomite, or other forms of calcium supplementation. They have the mistaken belief this will alleviate muscle cramps, menstrual pains, insomnia and nervousness. This is not true. Several enzymes see to it that optimum amounts of calcium are always in the body fluids. In deficiency it is the bones and the teeth that suffer.

The bones of Americans contain less than optimal amounts of calcium. As we get older our bones become increasingly demineralized, and almost all our elderly suffer from varying degrees of osteoporosis. The problem arises not from a calcium deficiency but from decreased absorption of calcium and from factors which cause minerals to be drawn from our bones.

When a fatty diet is consumed, the fats in the intestine combine with calcium to form insoluble compounds which cannot be absorbed. The diet of Americans contains an excessive amount of fat and this is undoubtedly a contributing factor in the development of osteoporosis.

Oxalic acid and phytic acid also combine with calcium to form calcium compounds that cannot be absorbed. Oxalic acid is found in high amounts in the following foods: beet leaves and roots, spinach, swiss chard, parsley, cocoa, peanuts, rhubarb, and wheat germ. Phytic acid is found in legumes and grains, especially in the germ and bran layers. Yeast contains an enzyme that breaks down phytic acid. Therefore, more calcium is absorbed when we eat yeast-raised breads than when we eat unleavened breads or grains in other forms. Phytic acid is also broken down when grains and legumes are soaked or sprouted.

Lack of vitamin D also results in decreased absorption of calcium. In the presence of sunlight, vitamin D is made in the skin. Then the vitamin is converted to its active form and carried to the cells of the intestine where it stimulates the absorption of calcium.

In considering osteoporosis we also have to look at factors that cause the calcium already in the body to be lost at an excessive rate. One important cause is lack of exercise. Exercise helps keep minerals in the bones, causing the skeleton to be denser and decreasing the risk of fractures. Lack of stress or weight-bearing movement causes bone resorption. Electrical stimulation is necessary for the proper functioning of bone-forming cells. Exercise that delivers rapid impact is most effective in generating the right kind of electrical signals to these cells. Walking and running are excellent exercises for this purpose. Weight-bearing exercises, such as weight lifting, are better than swimming.

When a person is bedridden, the skeleton bears no weight and the muscles rapidly lose nitrogen while the bones lose calcium. This is a problem the astronauts experience due to lack of gravity.

We lose minerals from our bones when we eat too many acid-forming and not enough base-forming foods. The mineral ash left in our bodies after our food is burned can form either acids or bases. When the body fluids are too acidic, minerals leave the bones to neutralize the acids. The acid- and base-forming foods are as follows:

Acid-Forming	Base-Forming	Neutral Ash
Meat	Fruits	Milk
Fats	Vegetables	
Eggs		
Grains		
Legumes		
Cheese		

The acid-forming minerals are phosphorus, chlorine and sulfur; the base-forming are calcium, iron, magnesium, potassium and sodium. A poor calcium-to-phosphorus ratio in the American diet is one of the main reasons for osteoporosis. The absolute calcium intake is not as important as the relationship between the two, there should be more calcium than phosphorus. The excessive consumption of meat is one of the factors contributing to this poor ratio because meat contains much more phosphorus than calcium. When we consume excessive amounts of protein and fats, calcium is lost in our urine. Eskimos, who eat even more fat and meat than we do, show significant bone loss at an even earlier age.

Natural means to protect our bones from significant calcium loss include:

- consuming yeast breads
- limiting foods high in oxalates
- spending a few minutes outdoors every day
- cutting down on meat and fats
- exercising regularly
- eating foods high in calcium
- increasing consumption of fruits and vegetables

The National Research Council recommends 800 mg. of calcium a day for adults. Many authorities feel this is more than we need. The World Health Organization recommends 400-500 mg. The following chart will show you how much calcium is contained in common foods so you can calculate how much you eat. It is relatively easy to obtain a sufficient quantity by eating a good diet.

DIETARY SOURCES OF CALCIUM

	Amount	Milligrams of Calcium
Skim Milk	1 cup	296
Broccoli	1 cup	136
Sweet Potato	1 large	72
Orange	1 medium	62
Apple	1 large	15
Apricots	3	18
Asparagus	1 cup	30
Banana	1	11
Cooked Legumes	1 cup	100
Green Beans	1 cup	62

Whole Wheat Bread	1 slice	25
Cooked Carrots	1 cup	51
Raw Carrots	1 whole	27
Cauliflower	1 cup	29
Celery	1 cup	27
Chicken	4 oz.	15
Cucumber	1 cup	26
Egg	1	27
Beef	4 oz.	13
Almonds	10	23
Haddock	4 oz.	11
Honey	1 tbs.	1
Lettuce	1 cup	19
Melon, musk	1 cup	23
Oatmeal	1 cup	22
Onions, chopped	1 cup	46
Green onions	1 cup	51
Orange	1	54
Oysters	1 cup	226
Peas	1 cup	38
Pizza	1 slice	144
Potato	1	15
Radish	1	2
Raisins	1 tbs.	6
Shrimp	1 medium	37
Spinach, cooked	1 cup	167
Winter Squash	1 cup	49
Sweet Potato	1	46
Tomato	1	15
Whole Wheat flour	1 cup	49
Non-fat yogurt	1 cup	300

People who take more calcium than their body needs excrete the excess in the feces. Suddenly discontinuing calcium supplements will lead to continued excretion of large amounts of calcium until the body adjusts to the lower level. In time the body adapts and becomes more efficient in calcium absorption. In many countries, calcium intake is much lower than our national average yet their children grow strong bones as long as they receive adequate sunlight.

During the last three months of pregnancy and during lactation women have an increased need for calcium. However, they also need more calories and their calcium needs should be met by the increased food intake.

More calcium will be absorbed if it is eaten at the same time as vitamin C. Certain acids keep calcium in a form that is readily absorbed by the body. Ascorbic acid—vitamin C—is one of these acids.

Phosphorus: Phosphorus was first isolated from urine in 1669. It glowed in the dark and ignited spontaneously on contact with oxygen; its name means "lightbearing."

Phosphorus is the tenth most abundent element in the earth's upper crust. As phosphate it is found in rocks, soils, oceans, rivers, and all living cells. Erosion causes the loss of phosphates from soil, especially sandy ones. We must replenish the soil with phosphate fertilizers in order to grow enough crops to feed the world's increasing population.

Phosphorus is the second most commonly occurring mineral in the body. It comprises 1% of the weight of the adult body—half as much as calcium. Ninety percent of it is combined with oxygen in the form of phosphates and is deposited in the bones and teeth. The rest is found in the cells of the body.

Phosphorus serves many essential functions. Phosphate is part of the genetic material in every cell, and it is part of ATP, the chemical form of energy produced from the food we eat. Phosphate also acts as a buffer for acids in the body. Excessive acidity causes phosphates and calcium to leave the bones to maintain the normal pH in the body's fluids. Some nutrients have to combine with phosphate in order to be absorbed through the cell membranes. Phosphates replace one of the fatty acids in the fat molecule to form phospholipids such as lecithin. The phospholipids transport fats and other lipids in the blood. Phosphate is part of numerous enzymes.

Phosphorus is a very essential mineral, but modern man gets too much. We eat large quantities of foods that contain a great deal of phosphorus in proportion to the amount of calcium they contain. There is an increased uptake of phosphorus in plants when too much phosphate fertilizer and pesticides are used. Phosphorus is also added to processed foods. It is added to ham to make it retain water and to cola drinks to give an acid taste. In this country we consume two to three times more phosphorus than calcium. This imbalance causes an over secretion of the parathyroid hormone contributing to excessive demineralization of bone.

We should try to decrease the amount of phosphorus ingested and increase the amount of calcium in order to maintain the proper proportion of these minerals in the body. This means increasing fruits and vegetables and decreasing protein foods in the diet. Cola drinks are one of the worst things we can consume as they contain large amounts of phosphoric acid. When your child loses a tooth, put it in a glass of cola overnight. You will be surprised to see the corrosive action on the tooth enamel.

Magnesium: Half the magnesium in the body is located in the skeleton, and it does not leave the bones as readily as calcium and phosphorus. The remaining magnesium serves many functions. It is necessary for nerve and muscle activity. It is an essential part of a large number of enzymes including those involved in the breakdown of carbohydrates, fat metabolism and protein synthesis. It is also necessary for the functioning of enzymes that convert energy to ATP. Magnesium is a fundamental part of more enzymes than any other mineral.

Magnesium is found in most unrefined foods, especially whole grains, legumes and vegetables. It is also found in large quantities in hard, but not soft, water. Fats, refined carbohydrates and alcohol contain very little.

People who live in soft water areas are more likely to be deficient in magnesium than those who live in hard water areas. In Canada and the United States, there is a correlation between the hardness of the water and the incidence of heart disease.

It is hypothesized that a magnesium deficiency is not manifested in blood levels of the mineral but rather in the heart muscle. The heart does not function properly unless there is an optimum number of magnesium and potassium ions. Deficiency of these minerals causes the heart to contract weakly and may result in irregular beating of the heart—arrhythmia. Arrhythmias are often the cause of sudden death. Magnesium deficiency is also one of the factors associated with atherosclerosis and with the formation of kidney stones.

Magnesium is found in abundance in whole foods but refining causes depletion. For example, the milling of white flour removes 86% of the magnesium from wheat. Refined foods not only replace magnesium-containing foods in the American diet, but also increase the need for the mineral because magnesium is needed to metabolize carbohydrates. Deficiency is not uncommon in alcoholics; symptoms are tremors and convulsion. Heavy drinkers, people whose diets contain a large proportion of refined foods, and those who drink soft water are apt to have low magnesium intakes.

Just as there is a calcium-to-phosphorus balance, there is a calcium-to-magnesium balance in the body. Calcium supplements not containing magnesium upset this balance, causing metabolic disturbances. As with calcium, low intakes of magnesium cause the body to be more efficient in its absorption of the mineral.

Potassium: The adult body contains half a pound of potassium, most of it inside the cells with a small amount in the fluid surrounding them. It aids in deriving energy from our food, transmitting nerve impulses, maintaining the acid-base balance in the body, and in the synthesis of protein and glycogen.

Potassium inside the cell exerts osmotic pressure preventing water loss. When excessive amounts of water are lost from the cells we are said to be dehydrated. Potassium deficiency can be caused by severe diarrhea, prolonged and excessive sweating, diabetic acidosis, and the use of laxatives and diuretics. Symptoms of deficiency are weakness, cardiac irregularities, respiratory and kidney failure. Extreme deficiency can cause death.

Potassium is found in most foods and it is not difficult to obtain sufficient quantities. However, excessive consumption of sodium will cause an imbalance in the body's sodium-to-potassium ratio.

Sodium: The adult body contains a quarter of a pound of sodium. Most of it exists in the fluid between the cells. Just as potassium works to maintain adequate fluid within the cell, sodium works to maintain adequate amounts of extra-cellular fluid. When sodium and potassium exist in the proper ratio, optimum amounts of fluid are maintained both inside and outside the cells. Like potassium sodium aids in maintaining the body's acid-base balance and in transmitting nerve impulses.

Sodium occurs in many foods and there is no problem in obtaining sufficient quantities. The problem is one of overconsumption due to excessive use of table salt—sodium chloride. We use it in cooking, we use it at the table and we use a great deal in processed foods. If no table salt were added to our diet, our daily sodium consumption would be equivalent to a teaspoon of salt. We get that much from the foods we eat. The American Heart Association says we need 0.2 grams of sodium, but Americans consume anywhere from 2.8 to 12 grams a day.

Excessive sodium consumption plays a role in causing high blood pressure—hypertension. When large amounts are consumed, the blood volume is increased. The blood vessels constrict in order to prevent too much fluid from leaving the blood, causing an increase in extracellular fluid. This results in hypertension.

An excess of sodium depletes the body of potassium. This in turn causes too much water to be drawn from the cells; it then accumulates in the fluid surrounding the cells. This is called edema, and is another cause of high blood pressure. One in five adult Americans has hypertension. It is a serious condition and is associated with heart disease, kidney failure and stroke. By the age of eighteen, 10% of American school children have borderline hypertension and their blood pressure increases as they get older. In societies where sodium intake is low, blood pressure is the same in old age as it is in early adulthood.

Epidemiological studies show primitive people with a low sodium intake have virtually no hypertension. In areas where especially large amounts of salt are consumed the incidence of the disease rises proportionally. Along the seacoast of Japan more salt is consumed than anywhere else in the world, and there is a proportionately higher incidence of strokes. On the Solomon Islands in the Pacific the coastal people use sea water for cooking and they experience a 10% incidence of hypertension. Further inland, food is steamed in fresh water and there is almost no hypertension.

There is a high sodium content in many foods, especially those of animal origin. People with hypertension may have to limit their intake of these foods. Other foods have large quantities of salt added in processing. These include butter, buttermilk, margarine, pretzels, potato chips, salted peanuts, olives, sauerkraut, frozen dinners, and processed meats—ham, bacon, frankfurters, salami and luncheon meats. Some pickles contain nearly a teaspoon of salt and some pasteurized cheeses contain twice the amount of salt as cheddar.

Soft water contains a lot of sodium. So do MSG (monosodium glutamate) and baking soda (soda bicarbonate). When reading labels look for salt, sodium Na (the chemical symbol for sodium), and soda. Hydrolyzed vegetable protein (HVP) is extremely high in sodium. HVP is often used for making vegetable broth and can be found in health food stores, advertised as salt-free. Avoid it if you want to stay away from sodium. Americans need to decrease the sodium and increase the potassium in their diet. We are eating more highly salted processed food and less fruits and vegetables. Our taste buds are used to salt. We become accustomed to it as infants because cow's milk contains three times more sodium than human milk. It is a good idea to breast feed babies for at least six months and to keep them off salted baby foods. At the time of this writing, Beechnut and Heinz have discontinued salt in their baby foods, but Gerber still adds it. It has been estimated that an infant fed commercial baby foods can take in eight times as much sodium as a breast-fed baby.

At first, getting used to unsalted foods presents a problem, especially for children. My advice is to cut down on salt gradually unless someone in your family has a health problem calling for a more sudden reduction. The local branch of the American Heart Association will gladly provide you with booklets giving cooking hints to make unsalted food more palatable.

People don't need to increase their consumption of salt during hot weather or strenuous workouts. Some sodium will be lost through the sweat. However, except in extraordinary situations of prolonged sweating, there is no need for extra salt. The body will adjust and begin to conserve more sodium if it is needed. Actually, potassium loss is more serious. The greatest concern regarding prolonged periods of profuse sweating should be with water loss. It is very important to replace this water. You can eat fruit or drink fruit juices to regain the water and the minerals lost.

Chloride: Chloride accounts for about 0.15 percent of the body's weight. The chloride ion is like potassium and sodium in that it helps preserve the body's fluid and acid-base balance. It is also necessary for the formation of a constituent of gastric juice—hydrochloric acid.

Chloride, like the other acid-forming minerals (sulfur and phosphorus), is found in abundance in meat, poultry, fish, eggs and grains. We obtain a good deal of this mineral from table salt. Since chloride is widely distributed in our foods there is no problem in obtaining sufficient amounts.

Sulfur: Sulfur is present in all animal and plant cells. Plants obtain sulfur in its oxidized form from the soil and incorporate it into organic compounds which can be used by animals. It is part of thiamin, pantothenic acid, and biotin. It is also part of three amino acids—methionine, cystine and cysteine. It is, therefore, found in high amounts in protein foods. Our requirement for sulfur can be met by obtaining adequate amounts of methionine. Legumes are one very rich source of this amino acid.

Sulfur is present in large amounts in the proteins of hair, nails and skin. The sulfur atoms of one protein molecule can join with those of another protein molecule giving strength to these tissues. Diets containing ample amounts of protein and the essential amino acids provide adequate amounts of sulfur.

TRACE MINERALS

In addition to the seven macronutrient minerals discussed above, there are many minerals occurring in the body in relatively small amounts. They are referred to as trace minerals.

Iron: We are probably more familiar with iron than any other trace mineral. It is the same substance from which your cast iron skillet is made. There are only four grams of iron in the body but it serves a vital function. The red cells of our blood are filled with hemoglobin. Iron, part of the hemoglobin molecule, combines with oxygen in the lungs. The oxygen-rich blood is carried to the heart and is pumped to the cells of the body where the oxygen is released and waste products are picked up. In the cells the oxygen combines with the breakdown products of food, releasing energy. Without oxygen, no energy is released.

Iron is also found in muscle tissue where it serves to carry oxygen, and in enzymes which aid in extracting energy from the breakdown products of our food.

Iron-deficiency anemia results if dietary intake of iron is too low, if iron is not efficiently absorbed, or used properly. Anemia can also result from excessive blood loss due to hemorrhaging, heavy menstrual flow, or parasitic infection. The symptoms of anemia are fatigue and pallor, but it takes a physician to diagnose and prescribe for the condition.

The poor eating habits of industrialized man often cause him to obtain less than optimal amounts of iron. Many processed foods have been depleted of it, and all too often they displace nourishing foods in our diet. This is especially true of those who consume many sweets.

People in industrialized countries are more sedentary and eat less than more vigorous people in primitive societies. This leads to less than optimal iron nutriture. Teenagers are apt to be more deficient in this mineral because boys grow rapidly, and girls diet. Menstruating women can also be iron deficient because they lose iron each month. Women are more efficient in absorbing iron than men; if they receive an adequate diet they can make use of more iron. Men take in an average of 16 mg. of iron a day but only absorb 0.9 mg. Women, on the other hand, take in only 11 mg. a day but absorb 1.3 mg.

Iron in animal foods is somewhat more easily absorbed than that found in plants. Dairy products contain almost no iron. Organ meats such as heart and liver are very high in iron but should be avoided because of their high cholesterol content. Especially good plant sources are whole grains, legumes, nuts, potatoes, green leafy vegetables, apricots, peaches, grapes, plums, and blackstrap molasses. Iron is found in almost every natural food.

Only small amounts of iron are absorbed, and the type of food we eat has an effect on this absorption. Eating eggs along with iron-containing foods appears to decrease its absorption while vitamin C facilitates it.

The body is extremely efficient in its conservation of iron, which is stored in the liver and spleen. Red blood cells live for about four months. When they die the iron and the amino acids are released and recycled. The iron is carried to the bone marrow where it is used to make new hemoglobin.

Iron is retained in the body so well that it is possible to get too much. This happens in some African countries where only iron pots are used for cooking. This condition is called hemosiderosis; it is characterized by large quantities of iron stored in the organs. Hemosiderosis is not likely to occur in our country except in people with metabolic disorders or who take excessive amounts of iron supplements. Many infants have received toxic amounts from overzealous mothers who think that if a small amount of a supplement is good for their babies, larger amounts will be even better. Many women have also overdosed themselves with iron supplements. It is best to get iron from natural, unprocessed foods.

Cooking occasionally in iron pots is a good way to insure against iron-deficiency anemia. Don't be concerned if the pots rust a little; this isn't harmful and is apt to occur when you cook without oils or fats. However, the exclusive use of iron pots is apt to cause you to get too much iron. This is more liable to happen to men because they do not lose iron each month.

Zinc: There are about 2 g. or zinc in the body. It is part of about twenty enzymes; it is in insulin which controls carbohydrate metabolism; it is involved in the digestion of protein; zinc carries carbon dioxide in the blood; it helps form the nucleic acids from which the genetic material of the cells is made; and helps rid the body of lactic acid produced in the muscles during exercise.

Adequate zinc is essential for optimal healing to take place. Injury, surgery, and burns cause a redistribution of zinc from the blood into the liver. Zinc increases the rate of formation of new cells to replace those which have been destroyed. Many times zinc has been reported to improve healing of acne, gastric ulcers, ulcerative colitis, surgical wounds, burns, bed sores, and leg ulcers. There have also been reports contradicting these findings. It appears that taking zinc enhances the ability of the body to heal itself only when there is a deficiency of the mineral.

Zinc plays a role in combatting infection in four ways. It aids in increasing the stability of cell membranes, thereby helping provide a protective armor for the cell. It interferes with the reproductive processes of viruses. It increases the effectiveness of certain kinds of lymphocytes, the white blood cells that produce antibodies against foreign substances. And, it stimulates the activity of phagocytes, the scavenger cells that ingest invading bacteria. High levels of zinc, however, can depress this activity. Supplementation of zinc and other nutrients may be beneficial in the treatment of severe and prolonged infectious illnesses. During such illnesses, an increased amount of zinc is lost in the urine, sweat, and probably in the stool.

Severe zinc deficiency results in decreased growth, loss of appetite, hair loss, skin lesions, impaired reproductive functions, poor wound healing, and an impaired sense of taste. The RDA for zinc is 15 mg. a day. The average American diet contains about 10 mg. Some people think the RDA level for zinc is set too high. If you make the dietary changes recommended in this book, you will obtain sufficient zinc.

In the 1960s it was discovered that 3% of the inhabitants of rural villages in Iran, Egypt and other Middle East countries suffered from adolescent dwarfism. Zinc deficiency was the cause. The diet of these rural people was high in unleavened bread containing large amounts of phytic acid which inhibit absorption of zinc and other minerals. Because of the hot climate zinc was also lost through excessive sweating. And many of the sufferers had snail fever, a disease caused by a parasite inhabiting the circulatory system. All these factors contributed to zinc deficiency.

Overconsumption of zinc through mineral supplementation can lead to several problems. There is a zinc-copper ratio in the body; if the zinc is too high it results in high levels of cholesterol in the blood and increased mortality from heart disease. A zinc-supplemented diet is thought to accelerate the development of some kinds of cancer. Too, taking high levels of zinc will cause a deficiency of selenium. Sometimes taking excessive amounts of zinc results in symptoms resembling those seen in zinc deficiency.

Copper: There are only 80 to 100 mg. of copper in the human body. Its presence is necessary for the release of iron stored in the liver which is then used in the formation of hemoglobin. In addition, it plays a role in the release of energy; it is necessary for the strength of body tissues; it is required to form the pigment in hair and skin; and it is required for formation of phospholipids.

Copper is found in abundance in whole grains, legumes, nuts, and grapes. Milk and vegetables do not contain much.

Copper is mainly excreted in the feces. Deficiency causes a decrease in the rate of growth, a loss of appetite, loss of hair color and anemia. Deficiency of copper has been reported in humans only in the presence of certain diseases causing an impairment of copper absorption.

Copper deficiency is very rare in this country. The problem is the relative proportion of copper to other minerals. Imbalance can be brought about by the consumption of soft water run through copper tubing which can cause the water to contain excessive amounts of copper. Imbalances can also be the result of inborn errors of metabolism. It is thought, for instance, that certain types of schizophrenia are caused by the combination of zinc and manganese deficiency with a relative increase in iron and/or copper. Such metabolic diseases should be treated only by a competent physician. Imbalances can also result from the indiscriminate use of mineral supplements. Some people express concern that we may not be getting optimal amounts of the mineral selenium. Yet taking zinc and copper supplements increase the need for this mineral.

Selenium: Selenium is physically and chemically similar to sulfur. Like vitamin E, it acts as an antioxidant. Selenium deficiency has been found to increases the risk of cancer. Deficiency has not been seen in this country although it does exist in certain areas of China.

Supplementation advocates say we should include this element in our diet to prevent cancer and to cure a host of other illnesses. They say, and it is true, the soil in some areas contains very little selenium, while the soil in other areas is rich in the mineral. Some areas are, in fact, so rich in selenium that it accumulates in toxic amounts in certain kinds of plants eaten by livestock. Many animals of the Great Plains have been lost because of selenium toxicity. It causes "alkali disease" and "blind staggers." Plants eaten by humans do not accumulate selenium in such excessive amounts. However, grains and vegetables grown in some parts of our country contain less than optimal amounts while those grown in other areas contain more. Because we find food in our markets that has been grown all over the United States, it generally balances out.

Selenium should be obtained only from foods since supplements can cause toxicity. When it exists in the body in large amounts, it interferes with reactions involving sulfur.

Rich sources of selenium are fish and whole grains. Good sources are garlic, mushrooms, asparagus, radishes, cabbage, onions, carrots, meat and milk. In addition to eating these foods, care should be taken to obtain adequate amounts of vitamin E since it may serve many similar functions. Zinc and copper supplementation should be avoided as increased levels of these minerals will increase the need for selenium. Always remember it is exceedingly easy to upset the intricate and delicate balance the body maintains.

Iodide: Iodide is no longer of great concern in the U.S. but it was in the early 1900s. The soil in the Midwest and the Great Lakes area is deficient in iodide-containing compounds. These areas are referred to as the Goiter Belt. Before the wide distribution of foods, people living in these areas developed goiters (enlarged thyroid glands) in epidemic numbers. A high incidence of goiters was seen in mountainous areas all over the world, including the Pyrenees, Alps, Himalayas, Sierras, Andes and Carpathians.

The thyroid gland is located in the neck next to the windpipe. This gland produces an iodide-containing hormone, thyroxine, which controls the rate of metabolism. When insufficient quantities are present, the thyroid gland works harder in its attempt to produce the necessary hormone and this causes goiter. The absence of sufficient thyroxine results in hypothyroidism or myxedema. People with this condition tend to be overweight, lethargic, have dry skin, a sensitivity to cold, and husky voices. If a woman suffers a severe iodide deficiency during pregnancy, she can give birth to a cretin. Such children are stunted in both physical and mental development.

People in the United States no longer suffer from iodide deficiencies because potassium iodide is now added to table salt, and produce in our markets comes from all areas of the country. Deep ocean fish are a rich source of this mineral; however, fresh water fish contain little.

Manganese: Manganese, like calcium and phosphorus, is needed for normal bone development. It is also part of an enzyme needed to transform the waste products of protein metabolism into urea. Whole grains and legumes are good sources of this mineral and it is also found in many vegetables. Animal products do not contain much manganese. Almost all diets contain an ample supply.

Toxicity has only been seen in miners who inhale large quantities of manganese dust.

Chromium: Chromium plays a role in carbohydrate metabolism. It interacts with insulin at the cell wall and facilitates the movement of glucose from the blood into tissue cells where it can be metabolized. Too much chromium, however, has the opposite effect. Chromium also plays a role in lipid and protein metabolism and deficiency has been implicated in the development of atherosclerosis. Good sources of this mineral are whole grains, meat, poultry and milk. The consumption of large amounts of sugar and refined grains may lead to a deficiency.

Cobalt: Cobalt is important because it is part of the vitamin B_{12} molecule. In the absence of cobalt, bacteria cannot synthesize this vitamin. Cobalt is necessary for the activation of several enzymes and may be capable of replacing zinc in others. Cobalt in foods is only of use to man if it is part of the B_{12} molecule.

Toxicity was seen in men drinking large amounts of beer to which cobalt had been added to prevent formation of excessive foam. They developed congestive heart failure.

Fluoride: Fluoride-containing compounds are abundant in the earth's crust. The amount of fluoride in the soil increases with depth, and the soil in some areas, e.g. the Dakotas, contains more than in other areas. Natural waters differ greatly in the amount they contain, depending on their source. Water from rivers and lakes usually contains less than spring and well water. The coastal areas of the Northeast contain an average of 0.02 to 0.1 ppm (parts per million). In the West, Midwest and South the water contains about 0.2 ppm. In some places the concentration in water is as high as 2 to 7 ppm and in these areas there is a high incidence of tooth mottling. Excess fluoride can be removed chemically and less mottling occurs at 1 ppm.

Almost all plants consumed by man contain fluoride but in small amounts since they absorb little even when the soil content is high. Food from plant and animal sources contains about the same amount, except for seafood which is high in fluoride. In addition to water and food, the air is also a minor source of fluoride. Both atmospheric pollution and humidity increase the amount of fluoride we obtain from the air.

The amount of fluoride in the body is very small and 99% of it is found in the bones and teeth. Fluoride has an inhibitory effect on many enzymes but increasing the fluoride intake of a population decreases the incidence of tooth decay. In many cities, fluoride is added to the water supply to bring the content to 1 ppm. This amount is within the optimal range. It should be borne in mind that healthy teeth are dependent on many factors and fluoride supplementation is no guarantee that decay will be prevented. There are many people with low fluoride intake and very sound teeth.

As with any other substance, huge doses of fluoride will result in toxicity or even death.

Fluoride in conjunction with calcium supplementation is sometimes used in the treatment of osteoporosis in the elderly. The pros and cons of this type of treatment are still under investigation.

Molybdenum: It has not yet been proven that molybdenum is an essential mineral for man, although it is found in small amounts in our tissues. The mineral is necessary for animals and it probably is for man. It is part of an enzyme which can play a role in the formation of uric acid, but it is not essential. The mineral is readily absorbed from the intestinal tract and just as readily excreted in the urine. An increase in dietary copper increases the rate of excretion. For this reason, copper is given to cattle who have fed on plants grown in soil containing excessive amounts of molybdenum.

Silicon: Silicon has recently been added to the list of essential minerals, although the amount needed is not yet known. It is necessary for the calcification of bone and the integrity of the support tissues of the body. It is also important for the growth of hair and nails. Man obtains most of his silicon intake from foods of plant origin.

Tin: Tin is found in many of the foods we eat and in many of our tissues. It is essential for the growth of rats but too little is known about whether it is needed by man.

Nickel and Vanadium: These two minerals have been found to be essential for man but their function is not well understood.

In the future other minerals may be found to be essential. Possible candidates are bromide and boron—the latter is definitely necessary for plants. Some minerals are used in medicine (e.g. lithium in the treatment of certain mental disorders) but this does not necessarily mean they are essential nutrients.

HEAVY METALS

Some minerals contaminating the food supply of industrialized civilizations are toxic to man. They are referred to as heavy metals and include lead, mercury, cadmium and arsenic.

Lead: Lead is present in the atmosphere from lead-containing fuels, industry, and cigarette smoke. Lesser amounts of lead are found in the tissues of people who live in rural areas. However, diet is the major source of lead in man and most of this is contributed by lead solder in canned foods. Some foods are contaminated by lead-containing pesticides, but this is not a large factor in lead contamination. Foods grown close to highways contain more lead than do those grown further away, but the contribution of atmospheric lead to the plants isn't very great.

More than 90% of the lead in the body is located in the skeleton. Contemporary American skeletons contain 500 times more lead than those of Peruvian Indians living 1800 years ago. Lead interferes with the action of several enzymes. Ingestion of excessive amounts causes anemia, nerve and brain damage, severe abdominal pain, occasionally gout and blindness. Symptoms of lead poisoning include headaches, insomnia, depression, and irritability. Sometimes twitching movements or tremors are experienced, and occasionally seizures. Some researchers think lead is a cancer-causing agent.

Lead poisoning is often seen in people who consume large amounts of illegal liquor because stills are put together with lead solder. In the past, it was not uncommon for children to be poisoned by chewing on toys, furniture or window sills painted with lead-based paints.

Fatal poisoning has also occurred in people who use lead-glazed earthenware pottery purchased in Mexico or Canada. It is dangerous to use this type of pottery for acidic foods or beverages. The risk of toxicity increases if these substances remain in the pottery for extended periods.

Mexican pottery is very beautiful and you can make it safe. The New Mexico State Health Department recommends washing your pottery thoroughly in soap and water. Rinse. Fill with vinegar and let it sit overnight. Pour out the vinegar, wash and rinse again. Other sources of lead include silver-plated vessels, porcelain pots and pans, pewter, and leaded crystal.

We are not the first people to have poisoned ourselves with lead. In ancient Rome, the aristocracy used plates and vessels made from lead, a rare metal used only by the rich. It has been found that Roman bones contain large amounts of lead. This is thought to be why so few children were born to these people and why so many died young.

The major source of lead contamination in our food is the solder used in the seams of cans. It accounts for half the lead in our diet. The Food and Drug Administration and other governmental agencies are working on ways to reduce this problem. Coloring agents and other additives can also be sources of lead.

Mercury: Mercury is extremely toxic. Ingested mercury compounds accumulate in the kidneys. It causes lack of coordination, confusion, and often death. Chemical plants sometimes dump mercury-containing wastes into waters thereby polluting the fish. Deep ocean fish are freer of contamination than are those closer to the shore. Deep ocean fish include red snapper, halibut, flounder and haddock. Larger fish should be avoided since they are at the top of the food chain and accumulate all the toxins ingested by the smaller ones. The largest amounts of mercury have been found in tuna.

In the early 1960s Japanese fishermen around Minamata bay were severely poisoned with mercury from industrial wastes dumped in the bay. Detective work finally pinpointed the cause but not before many people succumbed to this pollution.

Cadmium: Cadmium is found in minute amounts in the tissues of most animals, especially in the kidneys, and may play a role in normal human metabolic processes. It is not well absorbed and is excreted slowly. It might lead to the development of hypertension, especially when there is a high cadmium-to-zinc ratio in the body. It produces abnormalities in the arterial wall and also causes the body to retain sodium. In addition, cadmium causes damage to the pancreas and interferes with carbohydrate metabolism. Refined grains have been depleted of zinc and therefore contain a high cadmium-to-zinc ratio. High amounts of cadmium are found in rivers subject to industrial dumping from zinc smelters or factories producing cadmium nickel batteries. It is also in soft tap water and cigarette smoke.

Arsenic: Arsenic is another heavy metal contaminant. It is used in pesticides and weedkillers. It is also found in fairly large amounts in seafood. In spite of its reputation, it is relatively innocuous to man.

DRUGS AND MINERALS

As with vitamins, drugs can affect mineral nutriture. Diuretics (water pills) cause the body to lose potassium, and are especially dangerous if the patient is also taking digitalis. Aluminum-containing antacids can inhibit the absorption of phosphorus and fluoride and increase the excretion of calcium. Oral contraceptives can increase the need for several minerals. If you are taking any kind of medication including those that can be bought over the counter, you should check with your doctor to learn the nutritional implications.

Chapter 10

ALCOHOL

Alcohol is devoid of carbohydrates, fats, protein, fiber, vitamins, or minerals. It is considered a food because, like refined sugar, it contains many calories. In fact, whereas sugar consists of four calories per gram, alcohol consists of seven. Alcohol is considered a drug because of its potent effect on the brain, the nervous system, the muscles (including the heart), the liver, the circulatory system, and the endocrine system (the glands that secrete hormones). It is a much abused drug in our country.

Alcohol is highly toxic. The toxicity of drugs is described in terms of therapeutic index. This is the ratio of the lethal dose to the median effective dose. The higher the therapeutic index, the safer the drug is considered. For secobarbital, a barbiturate, the therapeutic index is 20. For alcohol (ethyl alcohol) it is 8. In other words, ethyl alcohol is 2½ times more dangerous than the barbiturate. These figures are approximate since the effect will vary from individual to individual and for the same individual from day to day. However, the amount commonly drunk is dangerously close to the lethal dose. Alcohol poisoning can result from a single binge and lead to death. Combining alcohol with other drugs, especially tranquilizers, will cause a depression of cardiac function and respiration, greatly increasing the risk of fatality. Just one or two drinks can have serious consequences when combined with some drugs.

Alcohol is absorbed extremely rapidly. In fact, quite a bit is absorbed before it reaches the intestines since it is readily absorbed in the mouth, esophagus, and stomach. It is absorbed faster in 10-20% dilution, as in wines and cocktails. In greater concentration, it is irritating to the mucous lining of the digestive tract inhibiting absorption.

Alcohol affects mental activities first and then motor activities. It is a sedative or calming agent. People are apt to self-medicate with alcohol when they are upset, when they are hungry, or when they are overstimulated from excessive coffee drinking. A breakdown product of alcohol, acetaldehyde, is a hypnotic (induces sleep). However, it interferes with dream sleep and can worsen insomnia. It also raises blood pressure and causes nausea, vomiting, and sweating. Alcohol depresses the central nervous system and is very dangerous in combination with other depressants. Stimulants, e.g. coffee, don't cause alcohol to be metabolized faster. They sometimes help counteract the drowsiness caused by alcohol, but they can worsen the situation.

Alcohol is also a diuretic causing the excretion of a large volume of dilute urine. For this reason, hangovers are characterized by excessive thirst.

THE LIVER

There are many alcohols, but the term commonly refers to ethanol—ethyl alcohol—a waste product of the fermentation of carbohydrate by yeasts or bacteria. Alcohol is a very small molecule, containing only two carbon atoms. It is oxidized only in the liver and the liver is the first and main organ in the body to suffer the consequences of over-indulgence. The liver is vital to our well-being. It manufactures more than a thousand different enzymes. It processes nutrients absorbed from the intestine before they are released into the general circulation. The liver produces special substances enabling the blood to clot when necessary. It makes bile which emulsifies fats so they can be digested by intestinal enzymes. The liver removes and neutralizes toxic substances from the blood.

Alcohol is detoxified by the liver, but this occurs very slowly. It takes two hours for the alcohol in one drink to be metabolized. If you consume more than one drink every two hours, the alcohol will affect your brain causing intoxication. The liver also produces antibodies. Large amounts of alcohol impair this function increasing the susceptibility to infection.

It is easier to catch a cold after going on a bender!

In the liver, an enzyme called alcohol dehydrogenase catalyzes the conversion of alcohol to acetaldehyde by removing two hydrogen atoms. It is the acetaldehyde that is thought to cause alcohol to be addictive just as it is the nicotine in cigarettes that causes people to become addicted to smoking.

Alcohol Metabolism

Drinking on a regular basis results in liver damage from a deposition of fats. The fat droplets accumulate in the liver cells. They coalesce as they increase in number, forming large globules up to four times their original size. There are three stages of liver damage.

Fatty liver is the first stage of injury. It can be the result of "moderate" drinking—one or two drinks a day—especially if a person is poorly nourished. If you are deficient in vitamins or eat a diet high in fat, there is a greater likelihood small amounts of alcohol will result in a fatty liver. This stage is reversible if the use of alcohol is discontinued.

If a person continues to drink, the condition will degenerate into alcohol hepatitis, an inflammation of the liver. This stage isn't easily reversed but cessation of drinking prevents further damage.

Cirrhosis is the third stage of liver damage. Fibrous scars form in the liver, the cells no longer function properly, and there is impaired circulation in the organ causing jaundice. Cirrhosis is the sixth leading cause of death in our country. It takes from 5 to 25 years for cirrhosis to develop. It occurs in 15-25 years in 25-50% of people who drink 5½ oz. of alcohol a day.

HYPOGLYCEMIA

There are many other adverse effects from the continued use of alcohol. Drinking has a tendency to cause hypoglycemia—low blood sugar. A molecule of alcohol contains many more hydrogen atoms in relation to the number of carbon and oxygen atoms than a molecule of carbohydrate, fat or protein. The excess hydrogen atoms cause a disturbance of the chemistry in liver cells. The liver rids itself of some of the hydrogen by forming lactic acid instead of glucose. This will result in low blood sugar, especially if a person is drinking and not eating. It can be fatal if the blood sugar levels drop to sufficiently low levels.

GOUT

In some people, drinking can cause attacks of gout. This is because the lactic acid formed when alcohol is metabolized competes with uric acid for excretion. When uric acid accumulates in the body, sodium urate crystals are deposited in the joints causing inflammation and pain.

HEART DISEASE

Preliminary research reports appeared in the newspapers recently stating that moderate drinking (one or two drinks a day) decreases the chances of a heart attack because it causes an increase in the amount of HDL cholesterol in the blood. However, as mentioned in the chapter on fats and lipids, some researchers believe that *total* cholesterol is a more reliable indicator of the risk of heart disease than the cholesterol fractions in the blood. While alcohol tends to raise HDL significantly, it has only a moderate effect on reducing the levels of LDL cholesterol. Therefore, the net effect is an increase in the *total* cholesterol in the blood. There is no evidence indicating that alcohol-induced higher levels of HDL afford protection against heart attacks. On the contrary, alcohol consumption contributes to the development of atherosclerosis and, therefore, to the risk of having a heart attack.

Some of the excess hydrogen atoms released during the metabolism of alcohol are used to form fatty acids which are quickly converted to fats—triglycerides. These fats are deposited in the liver and in the walls of the arteries.

In addition to causing the synthesis of fatty acids, alcohol inhibits their metabolism. It also causes the release in large amounts of hormones that stimulate the mobilization of fatty acids from adipose tissue. If a person already has atherosclerosis, alcohol will not only worsen the condition but is apt to cause kidney damage.

Alcohol also causes undesirable biochemical changes in the cells of the heart muscle causing it to function improperly. Heavy drinking, even if only occasional, can result in potentially lethal fibrillation, the rapid and ineffectual contractions of the heart. Hospital emergency rooms see this more frequently after weekend drinking and during the Christmas season; it is referred to as the "holiday heart syndrome." Occasional binges increase the risk of stroke in young adults free of heart disease. Adolescents are especially susceptible. In people with existing heart disease, a single drink increases the risk of stroke.

KETOSIS
Consuming large amounts of alcohol causes the formation of excessive fats and results in the dangerous accumulation of toxic ketone bodies. This condition, ketoacidosis, is seen in uncontrolled diabetics. It can result in coma and death.

HYPOXIA
Drinking results in hypoxia, a condition in which the cells of the body obtain less than normal amounts of oxygen. Oxygen is carried in the red blood cells. These cells travel through the capillaries, releasing oxygen to the body's cells. The release is facilitated by an enzyme system. Alcohol immobilizes these enzymes for up to twelve hours. Alcohol also causes the red cells to stick together preventing the transport of oxygen through the tiny capillaries. Brain cells are more affected by the lack of oxygen because their requirement is so high. Consequently we feel tired and our senses are dulled after drinking.

ULCERS
Although alcohol probably doesn't cause ulcers, it exacerbates the condition once it exists. This is because it stimulates the flow of gastric acids that irritate the stomach lining.

CANCER
Drinking significantly increases the risk of developing several kinds of cancer, including cancer of the tongue, mouth, pharynx, esophagus and

liver. If a person smokes, the risk is even higher. The incidence of rectal cancer is higher among beer drinkers. Alcoholics stand a much greater chance of getting liver cancer too.

While alcohol itself is carcinogenic, there are other cancer-causing substances in alcoholic beverages. For instance, beer, wine, and gin have been found to contain asbestos fibers. Beer also contains varying amounts of nitrosamines.

MALNUTRITION

Drinking contributes to malnutrition in several ways. Alcohol is high in calories, and often replaces nutritional foods in the diet. It causes inflammation of the stomach, intestines and pancreas resulting in malabsorption of many vitamins and of two minerals—calcium and iron. Mineral nutriture is also affected because alcohol causes the rapid excretion of magnesium, zinc, calcium and potassium. Alcohol also impairs the body's ability to properly utilize nutrients once they have been absorbed. Both alcohol and its breakdown product, acetaldehyde, interfere with the activation of vitamins by liver cells. This is especially true of thiamin. Added to this problem is the fact that the metabolism of acetaldehyde requires large quantities of thiamin further depleting the body stores. Symptoms of beriberi (the thiamin deficiency disease) are almost never seen in this country except in alcoholics. Thiamin deficiency is responsible for the tremors, psychosis and amnesia of alcoholics. Alcoholics often tell lies because they are terrified by their loss of memory and need to fabricate stories to fill in the time gaps.

In rats, thiamin deficiency will cause an increase in voluntary alcohol consumption. The drinking worsens the deficiency, causing additional drinking. Supplementation with thiamin may help break the cycle. Although I am generally against taking supplements, I believe in them for alcoholics. They should take vitamins of the B complex, especially thiamin. It has even been suggested, and not facetiously, that alcoholic beverages be supplemented with thiamin. Alcohol harms the body but some of the damage is caused by malnutrition; therefore, alcoholics should eat a proper diet and take vitamin supplements.

Forty-four percent of men and 27% of women who use alcohol are problem drinkers, or have potential problems with alcohol. Alcoholism involves more emotional and sociological factors than nutritional ones. What I want to stress is the habitual consumption of one or two servings of alcoholic beverages can have adverse effects on the body, especially in susceptible people. Unfortunately, there is no way of knowing who is susceptible and who isn't.

Large amounts of alcohol during pregnancy results in a much greater incidence of fetal alcohol syndrome (FAS). Children with FAS can be mentally retarded; some of them have facial abnormalities, whereas some merely gain weight and grow at a slower rate than normal infants. FAS is the third leading cause of birth defects. It can be prevented. In some women, the risk of giving birth to children with FAS is much greater when they drink moderately (two drinks) on a daily basis than when they drink heavily on occasion. Fortunately, alcohol becomes distasteful to some women when they are pregnant. According to Dr. Landesman-Dwyer, behavioral scientist at the University of Washington, the risk of affecting an unborn infant is approximately doubled by daily drinking an ounce of alcohol prior to or during pregnancy. There is 1 oz. of alcohol in 1 can of beer, a 5 oz. glass of dinner wine, or 1½ oz. of 86-proof liquor.

FEMINIZING EFFECTS ON MEN

Alcohol has undesirable effects on men also. It increases sexual desire but the ability to perform decreases. This isn't understood exactly although it may be related to a decreased level of testosterone, the male sex hormone. Alcoholic men lose masculine and gain feminine characteristics. There is less beard growth, the testes become softer and smaller, and infertility, sterility, loss of libido or impotence often result. Fat pads are found around the pelvic area and there is excessive development of the mammary glands which sometimes may even secrete milk.

MENTAL AND MOTOR SKILLS

Alcohol adversely affects cognitive skills and impairs memory. In some situations, men (but not women) have become more aggressive when they drink. Alcohol increases reaction time, affects coordination, peripheral vision and light adaptation, and impairs the ability to recover from glare, all of which have an adverse effect on the ability to drive safely. Nearly 60% of all traffic deaths involve a driver who has been drinking. The problem is worse when alcohol is combined with sedatives, antihistamines, or marijuana.

Alcohol is like sugar and oils; none of them is a whole food. Alcohol is the result of food processing, not by man, but by microorganisms. Whole foods contain cell walls and all the substances found within and between the cells. Alcohol, sugar, and oils are fiberless, partitioned substances that are rich sources of calories. They make a significant contribution to the development of the degenerative diseases affecting modern man.

Alcohol is a drug, a very potent and addictive one. No matter how little you consume, you are dependent on this drug if you drink every day. Combined with many other drugs, the action is greater than the sum of either the action of alcohol or the drug alone.

Because of the danger of addiction, because of the pharmacological actions of the drug, and because of the nutritional implications, alcohol should be drunk only occasionally. Alcohol should never be consumed for its physiological or emotional effects. To do so is to use it as a drug. Drinking a toast on New Year's is completely different from having a drink to help you relax. If you feel like having a drink when you are hungry, eat something instead. The craving will dissipate. People who are well-nourished don't have the craving for alcohol that mal-nourished people have. If you drink when you are tense; go for a brisk walk or jog. If you feel depressed, never drink alone. Try getting in touch with someone. Or take a walk. Exercise is an emotional normalizer. It picks you up when you are down and it calms you down when you are agitated. Exercise combats emotional extremes.

Take responsibility for your nutritional well-being and for your emotions as well. Don't submerge them in alcohol.

Chapter 11

BEVERAGES

What we drink is just as important as what we eat. I am going to discuss coffee first since it is the most popular American beverage.

COFFEE

Excessive coffee consumption is harmful because it contains caffeine. This substance stimulates the central nervous system and causes increased secretion of adrenaline. Drinking a lot of coffee causes an initial elevation of blood sugar followed by a period of hypoglycemia, and it causes an increase in lipids in the blood. Coffee can cause the heart to beat faster and sometimes irregularly ("skipped beats"). It causes constriction of the blood vessels and may raise the blood pressure somewhat. Therefore, people with hypoglycemia, those who are trying to lose weight, and those with heart disease shouldn't drink coffee.

Recent animal research has shown that coffee drinking during pregnancy can be harmful to the fetus. Caffeine increases the risk of cleft palate, missing digits, skull deformities and other birth defects. In recent studies sponsored by the National Coffee Association it was found that small doses of caffeine can cause birth defects in animals. The doses used were equivalent to a 100-pound woman consuming 4 to 5 cups of coffee per day.

Because the effects of caffeine were the same on chickens, rats, mice, rabbits and hamsters, it is predictable that humans are affected in a like manner. There have been several epidemiological studies on humans. In Belgium normal babies were compared with babies born with cleft palate, interventricular septal defect (an opening between the two sides of the heart), and other defects. The babies with birth defects were much more likely to have been born to mothers who drank 8 or more cups of coffee a day. Another study found women with a high intake of caffeine were more likely to have breech births, a greater number of miscarriages, and less active babies.

Caffeine is not only directly responsible for birth defects but it increases the birth-defect-causing effects of X-rays. It may also enhance the birth

163

defect potential of drugs, pollutants and other agents. According to the U.S. Food and Drug Administration, only a small fraction of a cup per day could be considered a safe level of coffee for a pregnant woman. Based on the data from animal studies, caffeine from coffee alone (not including caffeine from other sources) is responsible for thousands of defects in babies born every year in this country. In addition, experiments on male animals revealed that high doses of caffeine cause atrophy of the testicles and a lowered sperm count resulting in decreased fertility.

A preliminary study implicates caffeine intake with the development of fibrocystic and other benign (non-cancerous) breast disease. This problem is becoming more common among American women. The symptoms are lumps in the breast (usually the upper outer portion), soreness and sometimes discharge from the nipple. It becomes more severe just prior to the menstrual period. This disease is dangerous because it increases the risk of developing cancer and it can mask a malignancy, preventing its detection. It has been found that many women with benign breast disease drink large amounts of coffee or tea. When they gave up caffeine-containing beverages and chocolate, most of them experienced complete disappearance of the symptoms of their breast disease. Results were observed in some patients within a week. In younger women, it often required one to six months for the symptoms to completely disappear, depending on the amount of caffeine consumed and the sensitivity of the breast tissue. In women over 45, it took up to a year, probably due to the increased severity of the disease. Sometimes it was necessary for women to stop smoking in addition to eliminating caffeine from the diet. Those women who resumed coffee drinking had their symptoms return. A few were able to find a lower level of caffeine which did not result in the recurrence of symptoms. The surgeons who conducted this study recommend delaying biopsy or surgery in cases of suspected benign breast disease until caffeine has been eliminated for a while. Neither Mormons nor Seventh Day Adventists consume these beverages and their incidence of breast cancer is quite low.

Caffeine acts as a diuretic and can contribute to a deficiency of the water soluble vitamins. Coffee consumption increases the severity of preexisting ulcers because it causes an increase in the amount of hydrochloric acid in the stomach. Coffee has not, however, been found to cause ulcers. Caffeine consumption is often the cause of the restless leg syndrome. This is more apt to occur after a person has undergone gastric surgery.

In addition to caffeine, coffee contains various phenols. These substances are responsible for the aroma of coffee. Unfortunately, they act as catalysts in the formation of nitrosamines, which are known carcinogens.

Caffeine has many harmful effects on the body, and potent effects on the emotions. Caffeinism can cause a variety of mental symptoms which are not distinguishable from those of anxiety neurosis, including mood and sleep disturbances. Before investing large sums of money on psychiatric therapy for emotional problems, it would be sensible to abstain from caffeine. In many cases, this has brought a rapid and dramatic reversal of "instability" and emotional problems.

Cola drinks also contain a good deal of caffeine. Many pediatricians are concerned about children who drink soft drinks. They can become physically dependent on the stimulant and suffer withdrawal symptoms when it is abruptly given up. These symptoms include headache, anxiety, depression, sleepiness, nausea and cold sweats.

Coffee does contain a moderate amount of potassium, and a substance called trigonelline, which is converted to niacin during roasting. One cup of coffee provides 0.9 mg. of niacin. Since the RDA for niacin is 12-20 mg., depending on age and sex, you can see that this is not a significant contribution.

Coffee contains several undesirable ingredients including caffeine, various acids, a vasoconstrictor (constricts blood vessels), and mutagenic substances. Caffeine is the most objectionable of these ingredients. Different methods of preparing coffee result in varying amounts of caffeine in the brew. Instant coffee contains the least. Percolated and drip coffee have two or more times the caffeine. However, the amount depends on the brewing time and the grind, with more caffeine coming from the finest grind.

Many herb teas contain significant amounts of caffeine. Some blends, especially those with black tea or maté, can have as much or even more caffeine as coffee. Other caffeine-containing substances include cocoa and chocolate, numerous non-prescription drugs, and cola and pepper drinks. Some common drugs with caffeine are Anacin, Bromoseltzer, Cope, Midol, Vanquish, and Excedrin. Their caffeine content varies from 30 to over 60 mg. per tablet. Some carbonated beverages with caffeine are Coca-Cola, Dr. Pepper (regular and diet), Mountain Dew, Tab, Pepsi, RC Cola (regular and diet), and Diet-Rite. Their caffeine content varies from 32 to almost 65 mg. per 12 oz. can.

COFFEE SUBSTITUTES

Decaffeinated Coffee: Decaffeinated coffee is made from coffee beans which have had most of the caffeine removed. Formerly, the chemical trichlorethylene was used in the caffeine-removing process. However, it was found that in large doses, it caused liver cancer in mice and its use has been discontinued. Methylene chloride now is used and is presently being tested. Although decaffeinated coffee is almost completely lacking in caffeine, it still contains a vasoconstrictor. Decaffeinated coffee is, however, better for you than regular coffee.

Acid Free Coffee: There is an instant coffee on the market that is acid-free. It contains caffeine but most of the acids present in the coffee have been neutralized. The process causes less stomach upset and increases the potassium content of a cup of coffee to about that which is contained in a serving of orange juice.

Roasted Grain Beverages: There are instant coffee substitutes on the market made from roasted grains and vegetables. However, like coffee these substitutes have been roasted at very high temperatures giving them their dark brown color. Recent research indicates that excessive browning of foods causes the formation of mutagenic substances that may cause cancer. Nevertheless, these coffee substitutes such as Postum, Cafix and Pero are more desirable than either regular or decaffeinated coffee.

Here is a list of some possible effects of coffee and its ingredients: caffeine, phenols and acids.

- Increased secretion of adrenaline.
- Initial blood sugar increase followed by decrease.
- Increased blood lipids.
- Fast and irregular heartbeart.
- Constriction of blood vessels.
- Increased blood pressure.
- Harm to the fetus: cleft palate, missing digits, skull deformities.
- Increased incidence of breech births, miscarriages.
- Increased birth defect potential of x-rays, drugs, pollutants.
- Increased development of non-cancerous breast disease.
- Atrophy of the testicles.
- Lowered sperm count.
- Acts as a diuretic causing deficiency in water soluble vitamins.
- Increased severity of preexisting ulcers.
- Catalyzes the formation of nitrosamines.
- Causes mental and emotional problems and sleep disturbances.

TEA

Tea is a member of the camellia family. It is a tree that can grow to about 30 feet, but when cultivated it is pruned back to a small shrub.

Like coffee, tea contains caffeine, although in lesser amounts. Various brands of tea differ in their caffeine content. Generally, there is less caffeine in the brew when it is prepared from tea bags or from tea leaves in a metal container rather than from loose tea. The amount of caffeine ranges from about 20 to 45 mg. per cup in weak tea; in strong tea it ranges from 70 to 107 mg. per cup, depending on the brand and type of tea.

Tea contains not only caffeine but two related substances, theobromine and theophylline. Like caffeine, they are both stimulants. Theobromine is a heart stimulant. It also dilates coronary blood vessels and relaxes the involuntary muscles, such as those of the internal organs and blood vessels. Theophylline is a cardiac stimulant, a vasodilator, a diuretic and a smooth muscle relaxant.

Tea also contains tannins. These are the acids used in converting rawhide to leather. They are responsible for the "brisk" quality of tea. Their consumption is undesirable because they react with thiamin in the intestinal tract, preventing its absorption. Thiamin deficiency is not uncommon in Thailand where copious amounts of tea are drunk and fermented tea leaves are chewed. The tannins in tea inhibit the absorption of calcium, copper and iron. Tannins also interfere with the body's use of protein. Many studies have also implicated tannins in oral, esophageal and gastric cancer among those who drink large amounts of tea or among Asians who chew betel nuts which are also high in tannins. When milk is added to tea, the protein in milk binds the tannins and prevents them from causing as much harm. The English drink milk in their tea because they were warned of the danger of tannins by the British Medical Association. Ascorbic acid also inhibits the interaction between thiamin and tannic acid. If you don't care for milk in your tea, try it with lemon.

Here is a list of some possible effects of tea and its ingredients: caffeine, theobromine, theophylline and tannins.

- Caffeine related problems.

- Stimulates the heart muscle.

- Dilates the blood vessels.

- Relaxes the involuntary muscles.

- Interferes with the absorption of thiamin, calcium, copper and some iron.

- A factor in oral, esophageal and gastric cancer.

Tea from all over the world is from the same plant. However, it is processed in different ways. In black tea, the leaves are allowed to ferment. This reduces the astringency and develops the flavor and aroma. Green tea is prepared from unfermented leaves that retain their original color. Oolong teas, from Formosa and Foochow in China, are semi-fermented and the leaves turn a greenish-brown color.

The best quality tea is pekoe. Only the terminal bud and the first three tender leaves on the branch are used.

Tea is a fairly good source of manganese and fluoride. Because of the astringent properties of tannins, drinking tea can be helpful to a person suffering diarrhea. It is probably not as bad for you as coffee, especially since Americans like their tea weak.

HERB TEAS

Many varieties of herb teas are sold in health food stores and most people think that they are either harmless or good for you. However, there are bad as well as good effects from the use of different parts of plants. It is important to remember that not everything natural is beneficial. Infusions of the leaves, roots, flowers, bark and fruit of various plants have been used for centuries for therapeutic purposes. Herbalists have years of experience and knowledge passed down through the ages. In spite of this we are discovering habitual use of folk remedies can be harmful. The pharmacological effects of some plants are extremely powerful, and when they are used improperly, they can have adverse rather than beneficial effects.

There is a growing interest in this country in the use of herb teas to replace coffee. Because of ignorance of the potential harm of many of these herbal infusions, there are growing numbers of accidental poisoning. Reports of poisoning are appearing more frequently in medical journals. Some herbs responsible are pokeweed, pennyroyal, Jimson weed, ginseng, poke root and mistletoe.

Many herbs are harmless in small doses but toxic in larger amounts. Quite often it is a matter of common sense and moderation. Some people are experiencing adverse reactions because they drink enormous amounts of these teas when there would be no problem with occasional use. Some herbs sold commercially are contaminated with other unidentified and sometimes toxic plant material. This can occur accidentally when the herbs are gathered by those with little botanical knowledge; it also occurs when herbs are intentionally cut with other substances.

Ginseng, a member of the ivy family, is claimed to cure an almost endless list of ailments. Ginseng intoxication is referred to as the ginseng abuse syndrome. It causes stimulation of the central nervous system and can result in such symptoms as nervousness, sleeplessness, morning diarrhea, depression, and high blood pressure (although occasionally it causes low blood pressure). It also causes skin eruptions, edema and cessation of menstruation. Often, however, it is claimed as a cure for these conditions. Ginseng contains small amounts of estrogens and has been reported to cause sore and swollen breasts.

The root of the ginseng plant resembles the male genitals which may account for its popularity among the Chinese who attribute aphrodisiac properties to it. Ginseng tea twice a day and avoidance of sex for three months is a suggested cure for waning sexual appetite. It is very effective, since abstinence is probably the most potent aphrodisiac. Although ginseng is grown in this country, aficionados think the Korean variety is superior. Consequently, imported ginseng is very expensive and is often adulterated with potentially harmful plants, such as mandrake. Mandrake belongs to the nightshade family and has cathartic and narcotic properties.

Licorice root tea, in fact, licorice in any form, should be avoided by people with high blood pressure. It can cause the body to retain sodium and water and lose potassium resulting in an increase in blood pressure. In large amounts it can cause heart failure and cardiac arrest in susceptible people.

Like black tea, many herb teas, including maté, Lady's mantle, comfrey, Yellow Dock, Shave Grass and peppermint, contain large amounts of tannins. Comfrey, Yellow Dock and Shave Grass have been used in the tanning of leather. Yellow Dock also contains enough oxalates and nitrates that its consumption has resulted in the poisoning of grazing animals. Peppermint tea is effective in bringing relief from the discomfort of indigestion or gas pains. Its habitual use, though, will result in the ingestion of excessive amounts of tannins. If a person suffers from chronic indigestion or flatulence, he should seek the aid of a physician.

Alfalfa tea is touted in the popular herbal literature as a rich source of vitamins and minerals. However, scientific literature is full of demonstrations of its toxicity. Alfalfa is fairly high in saponins which cause bloat problems and respiratory failure in grazing animals; it contains a substance that inhibits the action of the protein-digesting enzyme, trypsin; and it interferes with the utilization of vitamin E.

Papaya tea has a cathartic effect and may cause abortion. It also acts as a depressant on the central nervous system and on cardiac function. Rose hips contain vitamin C but most of it can be lost during drying. The flower buds and leaves of senna contain potent cathartic substances and can cause severe—even fatal—diarrhea. Until recently many people drank sassafras tea. Because it contains safrole, which has been found to cause liver and other kinds of cancer, it has been withdrawn from the market. Safrole is no longer permitted as a flavoring agent in root beer and other beverages. Camomile contains only a small amount of tannins and is helpful in relieving indigestion. It was the tea given to Peter Rabbit after he escaped from Mr. McGregor's cabbage patch. Some people who are allergic to ragweed or goldenrod may, however, have reactions to camomile tea.

Unpleasant reactions are experienced by many people drinking teas made from unfamiliar plants. Some plants can be beneficial in the treatment of various conditions if properly utilized. There may be a place for the therapeutic use of herbs, but we need to increase our knowledge in this area. When herbs are used for medicinal purposes they should be supervised by a competent physician or practitioner.

Herbs can also be used in refreshing beverages. They should, however, be used in moderation until we know more about them. In the meantime, linden, camomile and Red Bush tea seem to be fairly safe. It would be prudent to avoid excessive consumption of more exotic herbs.

HERB TEAS

Generally Safe	O.K. in Small Amounts	Large Amounts May Cause Adverse Effects
Camomile	Maté	Pokeweed
Linden	Lady's Mantle	Pennyroyal
Red Bush	Comfrey	Jimson Weed
	Yellow Dock	Ginseng
	Shave Grass	Poke Root
	Peppermint	Mistletoe
	Alfalfa	Licorice Root
	Rose Hips	Sassafras
		Papaya
		Senna

Because many herb teas are potentially harmful, you should learn more about an herb before deciding to use it on a regular basis. I would suggest contacting either the American Medical Association for information or Dr. Julia Morton, a recognized authority on the pharmacology and toxicology of herbs.

The American Medical Association
525 North Dearborn Street
Chicago, Illinois 60610

Julia F. Morton, Ph.D.
Morton Collectanea
P.O. Box 248204
University of Miami
Coral Gables, Florida 33124

Dr. Morton has written a book called *Herbs and Spices*. If an herb is known to have a toxic constituent, it is mentioned here. It is available from Western Publishing Company in New York.

SOFT DRINKS

Soft drinks contain enormous amounts of sugar, artificial flavoring and coloring agents. Diet soft drinks contain artificial sweeteners that have caused bladder cancer in experimental animals. The cola and pepper-type drinks also contain hefty doses of caffeine. The combination of caffeine and sugar causes very erratic blood sugar levels, alternating from extreme highs to extreme lows. Some children drink enormous quantities of these beverages leading to hyperactivity.

In addition to all the other undesirable ingredients, soft drinks contain large amounts of sodium and phosphates. The excessive consumption of phosphates causes depletion of the body's calcium stores. (See *Protein* and *Minerals*) Phosphate shouldn't be added to the diet of a young person whose bones are growing at a rapid rate. Phosphates, too, are extremely corrosive to teeth.

Never serve soft drinks! There are many acceptable alternatives, including fruit juice and water.

ALCOHOLIC BEVERAGES

The effects on the body of alcohol are discussed in a separate chapter, but alcoholic beverages contain other substances, too.

Beer: Beer is made from fermented grain—usually barley—and from hops—the cones of a vine of the mulberry family. Some people think beer is a healthful, nourishing beverage. Actually, beer contains very few vitamins, most of them remain in the grain from which it is brewed. This nourishing grain is then fed to livestock. The brew contains a little calcium, phosphorus, sodium, and potassium. However, because alcohol is a diuretic, it actually causes a loss of minerals and can lead to deficiencies in magnesium, potassium and zinc, as well as the water-soluble vitamins.

Beer is quite fattening. The calories derive from alcohol and sugar. Although beer does not taste sweet, it contains maltose, a product of the fermentation of barley.

There is a correlation between how much beer is consumed and the incidence of rectal cancer. When the barley is roasted into malt, carcinogenic methylnitrosamines are formed. Nitrosamines are also found in bacon but they are not as toxic as those in beer. Different brands of beer contain different amounts of nitrosamines. In 1979 Coors beer was the only one free of these carcinogens since its barley is heated indirectly rather than kiln roasted. The other beers vary widely with some containing more than fifty times as many nitrosamines as others. Brewers are working on ways of reducing the amount of nitrosamines in beer.

Light beer contains somewhat fewer calories than regular. The alcohol content, however, is the same as that of regular beer.

A cold glass of beer may be a refreshing treat on a hot day; a couple of beers a day on a regular basis is not consistent with a lifestyle of moderation.

Wine: Wine is fermented grape juice. An antiseptic agent, usually sulfur dioxide, is added to prevent the growth of undesirable organisms, especially the bacteria that cause the formation of vinegar.

White wine is made from either green or black grapes. Red wine is made from black grapes; the juice is allowed to remain in contact with the skins long enough to obtain the desired color.

There is more tannin in red wine because it is concentrated in the skin. This is responsible for the characteristic astringent taste. In rosé, the juice is left in contact with the skins for a short period. The sugar in the various grape juices is converted by fermentative bacteria to alcohol and the gas, carbon dioxide. In champagne, carbon dioxide isn't allowed to escape, giving the characteristic bubbles. In some wines, carbon dioxide is added.

Some people think wine is a good source of B vitamins. It contains a fair amount of iron, converted by the fermenting bacteria to a readily absorbed form. Except for pyridoxine, however, it has a low vitamin content. Grapes are a better source of vitamins than either grape juice or wine.

Although wine contains little in the way of nutrients, it increases the absorption of minerals from food eaten with the wine. This is due to the natural acidity of wine and to the presence of certain non-alcoholic constituents. Experiments with zinfandel, an equivalent amount of ethyl alcohol, and dealcoholized zinfandel indicate the wine, whether it contains alcohol or not, increased absorption of calcium, phosphorus, and magnesium when it was drunk with meals. When zinfandel was drunk, the calcium absorption was doubled.

Wine has been served in some hospitals and nursing homes because it relaxed the patients and gave them a feeling of well-being thereby counteracting the effects of the institutional environment. Small amounts of alcohol, especially white wine, increase secretion of gastric juices, and wine is sometimes prescribed to stimulate the appetite in the sick and the elderly.

Dilute concentrations of alcohol cause a relaxation of the smooth muscles of the stomach and an increase in gastric motility. Larger amounts of alcohol, however, have the opposite effect. Red wine can cause a decrease in the amount of gastric juices secreted. The color of red wine, however, may have a beneficial placebo effect, enhancing the slight euphoria caused by alcohol.

Red wines contain somewhat higher amounts of methyl (wood) alcohol than white wine. Whereas ethyl alcohol is metabolized to acetaldehyde, methyl alcohol is converted to formaldehyde which is more toxic.

Red wines contain certain amines such as histamines and tyramines, which cause migraine headaches in susceptible people. Histamines are deactivated in the liver, but some people lack an enzyme (acetylase) which is necessary for this process.

Because alcohol stimulates the secretion of hydrochloric acid in the stomach, it should never be used by people with gastrointestinal disorders, such as ulcers, or any condition accompanied by hyperacidity. Wines are no exception—all forms of alcohol should be fastidiously avoided.

Some wines are contaminated with lead. Copper, lead or zinc are in some pesticides applied to vineyards. There is also lead in the exhaust fumes from cultivators. Another source of lead is the foil cap often used on better wines; it is 96-98% lead. Some wines are more acid than others and they will attack the foil if there is seepage around the cork and mouth of the bottle of aged wines. Wine bottles are stored on their sides to keep the corks moist. The porosity of the corks, especially those of inferior quality, can allow the wine to come into contact with the foil. If you observe a white powdery substance on the corroded foil, cork or mouth of the bottle, remove it carefully before decorking the wine. Then wipe the mouth of the bottle before pouring the wine.

Natural (unfortified) wines have an alcohol content of about 10 to 15%. Fermentation ceases at this level because this concentration of alcohol is toxic to the yeasts responsible for fermentation. Some wines are fortified by the addition of grape brandy. These include sherry, vermouth, Marsala, Madeira and port. They have a higher alcoholic content and are a good deal sweeter than natural wines. Their calorie content ranges from 34 to 49 calories per ounce, compared to 22 to 26 for table wines.

Dry (not sweet) white wines can enhance your cooking. They improve the flavor of such foods as sauces, casseroles and stews. Alcohol evaporates at 172 °F, quite a bit below the boiling point of water. When the alcohol cooks off, 85% of the calories will go with it but the flavor remains.

JUICES

Liquids enter the stomach faster than solids. Consequently, it is preferable to eat whole fruits and vegetables rather than to drink their juice. The cell walls of whole fruits and vegetables contain cellulose. Cellulose inhibits the speed at which the stomach empties its gastric contents into the small intestine. Once in the intestines, cellulose acts as a temporary barrier between the starches and sugars within the cell and the intestine's digestive enzymes. Therefore, they slow the rate at which carbohydrates are broken down and sugar is absorbed into the system. The juicing process breaks down the cell walls. If you drink fruit juice your blood sugar will, therefore, rise more quickly than if you eat whole fruit.

The lack of fiber in juice encourages overconsumption. Whereas a person would not eat more than one orange at a time, it is easy to consume half a dozen in the form of orange juice.

There is no such thing as a perfect food. No one food contains all the nutrients necessary to sustain life. And even completely unprocessed, natural foods often contain substances that can be harmful if consumed in large amounts. While vegetables contain many valuable nutrients and should be eaten every day, even they can be consumed in immoderate amounts if they are concentrated by the removal of fiber. There have been toxic reactions from the consumption of large amounts of vegetable juice. Vegetables grown under certain conditions contain high amounts of nitrates. If stored improperly the nitrates can be converted to potentially harmful nitrites, or they can be converted to nitrites in the body. This was the case with a two week old infant who was poisoned by carrot juice. He became cyanotic and irritable. This baby suffered no permanent harm because he was taken to a hospital fast enough.

Carrots, cabbage, spinach, melons, celery, lettuce and beets are apt to contain nitrates in large amounts, especially when they are organically grown. It is not a good idea to give young babies vegetable juices since their gastric contents are more alkaline. The alkalinity is conducive to the growth of microorganisms that can convert nitrates to nitrites. If infants are fed juice extracted from vegetables containing higher than normal amounts of nitrates or nitrites, methemglobinemia or the blue-baby syndrome may result. The baby's hemoglobin is prevented from carrying oxygen as with the infant fed carrot juice. If oxygen deprivation is severe enough, it can result in death. Acute toxicity is seen almost exclusively in infants.

Excessive consumption of carrot juice will yellow the skin, especially the palms, and the whites of the eyes. Carotenoids, which are yellow, will be stored in the skin when they are consumed in amounts greater than the body needs. Although this may detract from one's appearance, no other harm results. However, if a healthy person eats a well-balanced diet of natural foods, it is not necessary to obtain large amounts of vitamins and minerals from juices.

Fresh fruit or vegetables will quench your thirst. If children insist on something to drink, dilute their juice with water. However, undiluted juice is always preferable to soft drinks, especially those that are caffeinated. It is also better than whole milk with a high fat content; or chocolate milk which contains caffeine, fat and a large amount of sugar. If children are not too spoiled, they will drink the best thirst-quencher of all—water. Add a few slices of lemon to water and keep it in the refrigerator. This is a refreshing and healthful thirst quencher.

WATER

Sixty percent of the body is water. Most of it is in the cells and in the fluid that bathes the cells. It is in the blood, the lymph, the digestive juices, the bile, urine and feces. All the chemical reactions of the body can only occur in the presence of water. Water acts as a lubricant, reducing friction between moving parts of the body. It acts as a transportation system, carrying food, waste products and chemicals from one part of the body to another. Body temperature is regulated by loss of water from the lungs and in perspiration. Adults lose up to 6% of the water in their bodies each day. When you are sick or exercising strenuously, especially in hot weather, much more is lost. A 10% water loss is considered dangerous and 20% would result in death. It is important to replace the water lost from body fluids.

It is necessary to supply the body with large amounts of water but it is not always necessary to drink it. In fact, when adhering to certain kinds of diets, it is not necessary to drink any water at all. Water can be consumed in many forms, not only in beverages but also in the foods we eat. Fruits and vegetables are 75 to 90% water. Meat is 40 to 75%, and even dry cereals are 8 to 20% water. People on a diet of fruits and vegetables don't need to drink water. Chimpanzees in the wild have never been observed drinking water. However, people who eat meat need to drink water because more water is needed to rid the body of the waste products of protein metabolism.

It is important to drink water that is of good quality. You need to know about the kinds of water available so you can make healthy choices and so you will spend money wisely.

Purified Water: The water supplied by municipal systems is purified. It has undergone extensive processing to kill bacteria, remove viruses, and improve its appearance, taste and odor. While the spread of water-borne diseases has been very well controlled, new problems are arising and being dealt with. Chlorine added to water to kill disease-carrying bacteria can combine with organic matter from decaying vegetation and form harmful substances. These substances include chloroform, carbon tetrachloride, and many others. They have been found to cause cancer and other adverse effects. Methods to eliminate these substances are under investigation.

Soft and corrosive water can cause leaching of harmful minerals from public water mains and household plumbing. Although most of our intake of trace metals comes from food, harmful metals are sometimes found in our water. Lead is leached out of the soldering used to join copper piping, zinc from galvanized piping, and asbestos from asbestos cement pipes. A correlation has been found between the amount of asbestos in water and the incidence of certain kinds of cancer.Asbestos also occurs naturally in raw water in some areas. Our water is monitored for both naturally occurring substances and those that are a result of processing. The quality of this monitoring varies greatly, and new methods are constantly being sought to improve its quality. Check with your local water department and find out about the hardness of your water. Compare it against the standards of your county or state health department.

Hardness of Water: Water can be either hard or soft. It depends on many factors, such as the type of rock formation it passes through and the amount of rainfall. Hard water contains larger amounts of many minerals, especially calcium and magnesium. They can exist alone or as calcium or magnesium carbonate. Hard water has been found to be healthier than soft water because the minerals—calcium, magnesium, lithium, manganese, vanadium and chromium—act to protect against cardiovascular and other diseases. Soft water not only has smaller amounts of these protective minerals, but it leaches out more harmful metals from pipes and plumbing. These metals, if ingested, can alter the crucial mineral balance the body needs to maintain.

Populations living in areas with soft water experience more deaths due to cardiovascular disease. However, people find hard water undesirable because it leaves deposits on plumbing fixtures and causes problems with fittings, valves and equipment; it adversely affects the taste of the water; and soap is less soluble in hard water. Many people purchase water softening appliances that are plumbed directly into the water system. Water softeners contribute more sodium to the water. If the water in your house is softened, you shouldn't drink or cook with it. Have an extra faucet, outside the softening system, installed in your kitchen sink.

Some communities soften all the water. Fortunately, this is not often done. If it is in your area you can allow the water to run for a few minutes in the morning so the undesirable metals accumulated during the night are flushed out of the system. Or you can purchase bottled water.

Bottled Water: You can purchase spring water from nonindustrial areas in bottles. However, advertisements for spring water are misleading. Call the water company to find out what kind of water they supply to your area. One company in California provides spring water to the Los Angeles area but purified water to other areas.

Distilled water has had all the minerals removed. Some people think demineralized water tastes better, especially in cooking. Because of its lack of minerals it shouldn't be the only source of ingested water. Some distilled water has minerals added eliminating the problem. The chlorine compounds are not removed by simple distilling but they are in fractional distillation.

Mineral Waters: Mineral waters with a slice of lemon or mixed with small amounts of fruit juice are a nice substitute for alcoholic beverages. Some are carbonated either naturally or artifically. This carbonation can cause discomfort for people with digestive problems or hiatus hernia. The carbon dioxide, however, can exert an anesthetizing effect on the stomach and suppress nausea. Some bottled waters, such as Vichy, contain large amounts of sodium.

Buy mineral water if you enjoy it, but you will be wasting your money if you purchase it for its mineral content alone. Some kinds contain very little. The following chart will give you an idea of how much they vary in this respect.

Minerals in Bottled Water - mg. per liter

Brand	Calcium	Magnesium	Sodium	Potassium
Canada Dry Club Soda	63	11.5	243	6.0
Mountain Valley	70	7.5	4	1.0
Perrier	149	4.0	14	0.6
Poland	9	2.0	4	0.6
Schweppes	62	4.0	107	3.4
Vichy	107	11.0	1340	72.0

The above chart includes only a few of the minerals measured. To obtain the complete list you can write to:

California Department of Health Services
Food and Drug Section
714 P Street, Room 400
Sacramento, California 95814

For more information on bottled water, refer to a book on the subject by Arthur von Wiesenberger called *Oasis: The Complete Guide to Bottled Water Throughout the World*, Capra Press, Santa Barbara, Ca. 1978.

Home Purifiers: There are many home water purifiers on the market. Some use simple charcoal filters while other systems are very elaborate. The cheaper ones are not very effective and there can be a problem with bacterial growth in even the expensive ones. Distilling units are available but ordinary distilling does not remove all the chlorine compounds. Fractional distilling, however, does result in their removal.

Reverse osmosis systems, like distilling, cause the loss of most minerals, both harmful and beneficial. Most of the chlorine substances and pesticides, however, are also removed from the water. Before investing in a purifying unit, it would be worth your while to do some research at the library to make sure you are getting what you want.

The healthiest beverages available are usually the least expensive—water, fruit, and juices. Caffeine-containing beverages, whether bottled or brewed, and those that contain alcohol are highly undesirable when consumed in large amounts. Recent research shows that even moderate consumption of these beverages can be harmful to some people.

Chapter 12

SMOKING

Smoking has many harmful effects on the body. This is recognized by everyone with the possible exception of tobacco growers and the congressmen who are influenced by them. You may wonder, however, about the appropriateness of including a chapter on smoking in a book about nutrition. Smoking has a tremendous effect on the amount of oxygen that is supplied to the cells of the body.

Oxygen is an essential nutrient. We can't survive without it for more than a few minutes. It is necessary for the metabolism of the food we eat. Without it our food cannot be converted to the energy we need to stay alive.

In spite of the importance of oxygen, the body is very inefficient in obtaining it. Air contains 21% oxygen but the lungs can only extract a small proportion of that. A mere 10% of the oxygen we inhale is actually used by the cells. The rest is exhaled along with the carbon dioxide. The amount of oxygen available to the cells of the body is one of the most important criteria of good health. For this reason, a book on nutrition would be incomplete if it omitted a discussion of any substance that greatly decreases the availability of this important nutrient.

The toxin in cigarette smoke that relates directly to nutrition is the gas, carbon monoxide. It is the most harmful of all the ingredients of tobacco smoke. Do not confuse this poison with carbon dioxide, the waste product liberated in the cells during metabolism. Carbon monoxide (CO) has one oxygen molecule and carbon dioxide (CO_2) has two.

Carbon monoxide is the product of incomplete combustion. It is formed when anything burns and, therefore, is an ingredient of cigarette smoke. It combines two hundred times more readily with hemoglobin than oxygen does. This means it binds the hemoglobin so that it can't combine with oxygen. Carboxyhemoglobin is this combined form of hemoglobin. It is much more stable than oxyhemoglobin, and the carbon monoxide is not released easily but stays in the body for a long time. In addition, carbon monoxide inhibits the release of oxygen from oxyhemoglobin at the tissue level. Acute carbon monoxide poisoning results in death by suffocation—lack of oxygen. Therefore, a smoker suffers from partial suffocation.

Because it deprives all the cells of sufficient oxygen, smoking is implicated in a wide variety of diseases. Some cigarettes contain lower amounts of nicotine and tar but produce more noxious carbon monoxide. Cigars and pipes produce more carbon monoxide than do cigarettes. However, many cigar and pipe smokers do not inhale and are less likely than cigarette smokers to suffer from many of the adverse effects of smoking. When the smoke isn't inhaled, however, more carbon monoxide is released in the air to affect others.

SHOULD SMOKERS TAKE VITAMIN C SUPPLEMENTS?

Articles advising vitamin C supplementation for smokers have appeared in the press. It has been found that large amounts of vitamin C supplementation cause the smoker to lose more nicotine in the urine. Smokers, however, will smoke as many cigarettes as necessary to maintain nicotine at the level to which they are addicted. With more cigarettes the smoker is exposed to the same amount of nicotine but to larger amounts of other toxins in the smoke. If a person is unable, or unwilling, to give up smoking, some researchers believe it is best to use cigarettes high in nicotine so less are smoked. Exposure to carbon monoxide and other harmful ingredients will then be lower.

EFFECTS OF SMOKING ON THE BODY

Toxins in Cigarette Smoke: Smoking is harmful to the body in many other ways. Toxins in cigarette smoke include cyanide, phenols, aldehydes, acrolein, oxides of nitrogen and sulfur, ammonia, hydrogen sulfide, nitrosamines, nicotine and tar. Arsenic and lead are also found if insecticides containing these harmful metals were used on the tobacco crop. There are numerous other ingredients in cigarette smoke and they have many harmful effects on the body.

Lung Damage: Cigarette smoke contains free radicals, highly reactive substances that cause harmful changes to the lipids in the membranes of lung cells. Damage to their membranes causes impaired function in these cells and results in lowered immunity to infection by inhaled bacteria.

Other irritating substances in cigarette smoke cause abnormal changes in the delicate tissues of the lungs and bronchial tubes. Smoking is a major factor in the development of chronic bronchitis and emphysema, a condition in which the lungs lose their elasticity and the ability to inhale and exhale is impaired. People with smoker's cough (even very young smokers) are especially likely to develop these respiratory diseases. Almost all lung cancer in the United States is attributed to smoking. The consumption of alcoholic beverages increases the risk of lung cancer because alcohol acts as a solvent for the carcinogens in tobacco smoke.

Cardiovascular Damage: Smoking causes even more damage to the cardiovascular than to the respiratory system. It precipitates the deterioration and stiffening of small arteries supplying the heart with oxygen. These vessels then cannot expand to allow sufficient blood to reach the heart tissue. This can lead to an abnormal heart rhythm and often results in sudden death, which is twice as common in smokers. Nicotine stimulates the heart to beat faster at the same time it is deprived of oxygen.

Bone Damage: Smoking affects the health of the bones. There may be a relationship between smoking-induced atherosclerosis and osteoporosis. Smoking causes an increase in the acidity of bone tissue, in turn leading to mineral adsorption and porous bones.

Effect on Appearance: Smoking affects our appearance. It causes an increase in blood pressure and a narrowing of the small blood vessels in the skin. This results in less oxygen reaching the cells of the skin and is one of the causes of wrinkling. It also leads to cold fingers and toes.

Cancer and Birth Defects: Because carcinogenic compounds in tobacco tar are carried in the blood to all organs of the body, smoking can cause not only cancer of the lung, larynx, mouth and esophagus but also of the bladder, kidney, stomach and prostate. Smoking during pregnancy can impair the growth of the fetus because nicotine decreases uterine blood flow. Some researchers consider smoking to be the greatest hazard to unborn children.

Chapter 13

EXERCISE

Like smoking, exercise greatly affects the amount of oxygen received by the body's cells. The body responds in many ways to varying levels of activity or inactivity thereby affecting oxygen nutriture.

LUNG CAPACITY

The muscles of the rib cage expand and contract the chest cavity. With the cavity expanded, a partial vacuum is created in the lungs causing air to rush in. If the muscles do not work efficiently a limited amount of fresh air will come into the lungs and a limited amount of stale (deoxygenated) air will be expelled. Regular exercise strengthens the muscles of the rib cage enabling the body to take in more oxygen and allowing more carbon dioxide to be exhaled.

Vital capacity refers to the usable proportion of the lungs. The vital capacity of your lungs is determined by measuring the amount of air you can exhale after taking a deep breath; it is a simple test performed routinely by many physicians. The air remaining in the lungs after the greatest possible amount has been expelled is called residual air. If there is a lot of residual air, it means a large portion of the lungs is unusable. In this situation, a person will suffer from shortness of breath after even slight activity. Reduced vital capacity can be caused by weakness of the muscles of the rib cage. These muscles can be strengthened by exercise strenuous enough to induce heavy breathing. This is one of several ways exercise makes more oxygen available to the cells.

HEMOGLOBIN

The amount of oxygen entering the blood is limited by the number of red blood cells and the amount of hemoglobin in them. Exercise creates an extra demand for oxygen and, therefore, causes the body to adapt by producing both more red cells and more hemoglobin. When you exercise, you increase the oxygen- carrying power of your blood.

183

CARDIOVASCULAR BENEFITS

Exercise has a beneficial effect on the heart and blood vessels. Death rates from cardiovascular disease decrease with increasing amounts of exercise.

Exercise can increase the volume of blood by as much as a quart. It also increases the number of blood vessels so the extra blood can be carried to the tissues. More blood is carried to the skeletal muscles, thereby building endurance. More blood is also carried to the heart and a healthy heart is one with a good blood supply.

Exercise makes the heart larger and stronger and slows the pulse or heart rate. The heart of an unconditioned person is weak and pumps faster and less efficiently than the heart of a conditioned person. The heart rate of a person in good shape will be around 60/minute (or less) at rest; for one out of shape it will be 80/minute or more. A lower heart rate indicates a strong heart, one that beats less often but more effectively. It has more time to rest between beats. Although heart rate and blood pressure are elevated during exercise, a fit body has low resting rates. Exercise also stimulates fibrinolysis, whereby clots in the vessels are broken down preventing them from obstructing a small artery.

LIPIDS

Exercise lowers the level of triglycerides (fats) in the blood by increasing the amount burned or oxidized. Exercise also causes the body to make fewer fats.

Exercise will increase the amount of HDL cholesterol in the blood. This fraction of blood cholesterol may protect against heart disease; there is an inverse relationship between the level of HDL cholesterol and the death rate from cardiovascular disease. More people have heart attacks when their LDL cholesterol is high and the HDL cholesterol is low. Whether the exercise-induced increase in HDL cholesterol decreases the risk of sustaining a heart attack is controversial. Because of the many known cardiovascular benefits, however, exercise programs have been set up across the country for heart attack victims in order to decrease the risk of another attack.

VEINS

Contraction of the leg muscles gently squeezes the veins. This provides a pumping action that propels the blood along the veins. Exercise helps prevent stagnation and congestion of blood in these vessels. Some people think this congestion contributes to the development of varicose veins.

FATIGUE

Fatigue is caused by a lack of oxygen and an accumulation of carbon dioxide in the body. Exercise helps combat fatigue by bringing in more oxygen and quickly ridding the body of carbon dioxide.

OTHER BENEFITS OF EXERCISE

The most important effects of exercise are those related to the amount of oxygen taken to the cells. However, there are other benefits of exercise as well.

Emotional Benefits: There are emotional benefits to be derived from exercise, especially running or jogging. Exercise helps get rid of tension. Emotional stress causes the adrenal glands to produce hormones that in turn accelerate body processes. The alleviation of stress will result in less wear and tear by preventing the excessive production of these hormones.

There are many things people do to relieve stress. For example, they drink alcohol, overeat, smoke, or take drugs. Instead, try exercising!

Purdue University researchers were surprised to find that exercise helped develop a sense of self-confidence.

Jogging is effective in the relief of depression so common in our society. It also relieves anxiety and anger. Joggers know that if they have the blues, running for 30 to 60 minutes will help. There are psychological benefits from the rhythmical movement of the large muscles when they are not overtaxed.

Dr. John Greist and his associates observed that several of their moderately depressed patients made more improvement by increasing their physical activity than they did with psychotherapy. According to Dr. Greist, the more deconditioned people are, the more abnormal they will be psychologically. Physical activity can alter your mood and modify anxiety and depression. People feel better both during and after exercise, and it increases their work efficiency and improves their sleep. A group of 167 college students were evaluated before and after an eight week program of various types of exercise. There was no reduction in depression among the softball players and those who did not exercise. Depression was reduced in all the others, especially in those who jogged.

Dr. Greist recommends traditional therapies for people who are severely depressed. In those whose depression is mild or moderate, he recommends jogging because it is available to almost everyone, it is cheap, and it can be effective.

Biochemical changes occur in the body in response to jogging. During battle or in sports, often no pain is felt when a person is injured. Preliminary investigation by a group of researchers causes them to attribute this phenomenon to the production of opiates by the central nervous system.

Dr. Kostrubala, professor of clinical psychiatry, claims that slow, long-distance running is addictive. One who agrees with him is Dr. William Glasser, author of *Positive Addiction*. In his study of runners, Dr. Glasser has found that most of them suffer withdrawal symptoms if they are prevented from running. After running regularly for an extended period of time you may find yourself addicted. Some days you may have to push yourself to exercise. However, if circumstances should keep you from running for more than a couple of days you would be surprised at the discomfort and sense of deprivation and frustration you feel. Some people become so fond of running they let it take over to the exclusion of other things in their lives. It should be pleasurable but it should not be the only area of pleasure in your life.

The repetitive rhythm of jogging can have the same effect as chanting a mantra in meditation. The mind will turn off the ordinary world and lapses of time occur. Sometimes a creative idea or the solution to a problem will suddenly come to you. This effect is probably the reason people become addicted to running.

Even if you do not derive these esoteric benefits from your exercise program, it is infinitely valuable as a way of letting off steam.

Sleep: You sleep more soundly when you exercise. However, strenuous exercise immediately before retiring might prevent you from falling asleep quickly. Exercise often reduces the amount of sleep required and you feel less fatigue and more alert during waking hours. If the exercise is more strenuous than customary, you may need more sleep in the beginning.

Appearance: Exercise makes people look better. It slims the thighs and the fanny even when unaccompanied by weight loss. It firms the muscles and leads to better skin tone because of the increase in peripheral circulation. Long distance running prevents the loss of muscle tissue and the acquisition of fatty tissue that usually go with aging.

Weight Loss: People often experience a weight loss when they exercise regularly. You burn more calories when you exercise more than normally, but this is not the main factor causing you to lose weight. Instead there are metabolic changes caused by exercise. When sufficient oxygen is brought to the cells, more ATP—the chemical form of energy—is produced. There is always plenty of hydrogen in the cells, and when oxygen is in short supply, the breakdown products of food will combine with hydrogen instead of oxygen to form fats. Farmers and ranchers aware of this effect pen their animals to keep them inactive, thereby fattening them for market. Exercise also increases the secretion of adrenaline which in turn increases the rate of metabolism. Bringing more oxygen to the cells will cause you to be thinner and to have more energy.

Strenuous exercise has an appetite-suppressing effect. Researchers studying this effect in rats thought it was due to exercise-induced hormonal changes.

Even if you do not lose weight, exercise will cause a better distribution of the weight. It decreases the amount of "cellulite," the dimply adipose tissue of the thighs which plagues so many women and teenage girls.

Cathartic Effect: Among other benefits exercise has a laxative or cathartic effect because it stimulates the muscles that cause the intestinal contents to move.

Blood Sugar: Exercise is beneficial to diabetics because of its effect on glucose tolerance. It causes an increased consumption of glucose by exercising muscles, thereby lowering the level in the blood. Too, exercise effects the secretion of hormones involved with carbohydrate metabolism. Exercise also causes the insulin to be more effective in transporting glucose from the blood into tissue cells. An exercise program can be an important part of the treatment of most diabetics. It has been suggested that the recent decrease in physical activity along with adverse changes in diet are significant factors in the increasing incidence of this disease.

Diabetics who are taking insulin should make no changes in their level of physical activity unless they do so under the supervision of their physician. Exercise usually lowers excessively high blood sugar to normal levels. Occasionally, however, it can cause the blood sugar to drop *too* low. Marked hypoglycemia (low blood sugar) can occur in diabetics on insulin. It can also occur in some marathon runners, in people who are fasting, or in people who are on low carbohydrate diets.

Bone Strength: Exercise plays a very important role in preventing bone demineralization and the development of osteoporosis in older people. The stress on bones, however, must be great enough to cause an increase in their density. Running, walking and tennis are good exercises in this respect. Inactivity causes the body to excrete greater amounts of phosphorus and calcium, resulting in a weakening of the bones. Osteoporosis due to lack of exercise is considered a major health problem. (See *Minerals*.)

Gallstones: Animal and human studies show that exercise causes a lower concentration of cholesterol in the bile. Exercise makes the cholesterol more soluble in the bile preventing the formation of cholesterol gallstones.

Longevity: Aerobic exercise will increase your chance of living longer. Studies of British bus conductors and drivers, walking and driving mailmen, and longshoremen in Los Angeles have borne this out. The bus conductors and walking mailmen lived longer than bus drivers or mailmen who delivered mail in a truck. Among the longshoremen, those whose jobs required heavy physical activity had fewer heart attacks and lived longer than the ones whose work required less strenuous activity.

Insurance: Some companies are now offering life insurance policies at reduced rates to people engaged in a program of regular exercise. Contact your insurance company and see if it offers this discount.

TYPES OF EXERCISE

Not all forms of exercise are, however, equally beneficial. The different types of exercise fall into four categories.

Isometrics: Isometrics is exercise where there is contraction of the muscles but no movement. An example is pushing the heels of your hands against each other. Isometrics will cause an increase in the size and strength of individual muscles but this type of exercise does not create much demand for oxygen. People with hypertension should avoid isometric exercise, because it increases blood flow to the heart but not the pulse rate. This results in increased blood pressure and can be dangerous.

Isotonics: Isotonics includes weight lifting and calisthenics. In this type of exercise there is contraction of the involved muscles and movement, but no prolonged demand for oxygen. This type of exercise soon causes shortness of breath so the exercise is not sustained. To do the most good, the heart and respiratory rates must remain elevated for at least thirty minutes. Isotonics is beneficial for skeletal muscles, but not for the lungs, heart or blood vessels. Like isometric exercises, isotonics increases the blood pressure.

Anerobics: Anaerobics includes such activities as sprints and dashes, on foot or bicycle. These exercises do not create a long enough demand for oxygen to result in cardiovascular benefits. Short walks also fall into this category. Recreational bicycling does not ordinarily create a great enough increase in the heart or respiratory rate. Tennis is not as good as some exercises because of the intermittent rest periods between volleys; only a skilled player moves all the time.

Aerobics: The most beneficial type of exercise is called aerobics. This is rhythmic, repetitive activities involving the large muscles. It includes brisk and sustained walking, cycling upgrade for prolonged periods of time, stationary running, swimming, skating, handball, basketball, squash and aerobic dancing. These exercises must be sustained for half an hour to be beneficial. This type activity is strenuous enough to cause sufficient elevations of the heart and respiratory rates but not so strenuous that it cannot be sustained for a sufficient length of time. To be beneficial there must be a great enough demand for oxygen over a long enough period of time. This causes the body to adapt so that an increased supply of oxygen is brought to the cells. You should do aerobic exercises three times a week on nonconsecutive days for maximum benefit. For the aerotic benefits, the pulse rate must be sustained at a sufficiently elevated rate for a minimum of fifteen minutes. If the heart rate is allowed to drop before this, it will not give you the most important of benefits.

HOW TO START EXERCISING

When embarking on an exercise program after a period of inactivity, you should start out slowly. The degree of exertion should be increased gradually. It will take a while for the muscles, joints and other parts of the body to adapt to the point where they can withstand vigorous and prolonged exercise without sustaining injury. Until your muscles gain strength, they will limit the amount of exercise in which you are able to engage. Only when they have been conditioned, will you be able to carry the exercise to the point where your cardiovascular system benefits. Then you can sustain a sufficient elevation of the heart rate for a long enough period of time to be beneficial to the heart. You should exert yourself until you can feel your heart beating harder and until you are breathing more heavily but not to the point where you are short of breath. The best criterion in judging how far to go is how you feel. If you are too short of breath to carry on a conversation you should slow down.

For those who want to know what heart rate should be reached during exercise the National Jogging Association offers this advice. Subtract your age from 220. This number is an estimate of your maximum heart rate per minute. Multiply by 0.70 if you *have not* been jogging regularly, 0.75 if you *have*, and 0.65 if you smoke more than 6 cigarettes a day or if you are more than 20 pounds overweight. Don't count weight gain during pregnancy. The resulting number is the number of times per minute your heart should be able to beat safely and still provide you with aerobic benefits. Divide this number by 6. This is the number of heart beats you should count when you interrupt your exercise to take your pulse for 10 seconds. At rest it is more accurate to take your pulse for 15 seconds and multiply by 4 to see how many times it beats in a minute. When you stop exercising, however, your heart rate slows down so rapidly that counting it for 15 seconds would be less accurate.

For instance, if you are 45 years of age and have been engaged in a regular program of exercise, you would figure your target heart rate in the following manner:

$$220 - 45 \text{ (age)} = 175$$

$$175 \times .75 = 131 \text{(target heart rate/minute)}$$

$$131 \div 6 = 22 \text{(target heart rate/10 seconds)}$$

Don't tax yourself when you are starting out because your blood vessels may be in worse shape than you realize. If you are immoderate, you could precipitate a heart attack. Men over 35 should always check with their physician before engaging in any exercise program. Before menopause, women are less at risk of developing cardiovascular disease as they are partially protected by their higher levels of estrogen. However, after menopause, they also should consult with their physician to determine their exercise tolerance; as should people of any age who are obese. Even if you are young and not overweight, if you have been eating a high fat diet for a long period of time, vigorous exercise may do you more harm than good. It would be better to adhere to a program of walking and consult with your physician before engaging in more strenuous kinds of exercise.

He may decide to test for undiagnosed heart disease. Fifteen to 20% of Americans have heart disease without knowing it.

You should choose a type of exercise you enjoy or it will be difficult to stick with it. Choose one (or more) you will be able to fit into your schedule and one that is compatible with your lifestyle. Whatever exercise you choose, make sure you have the proper equipment for it. For walking or jogging buy a proper pair of shoes. They need not be expensive but they must be especially made for your activity, must fit well, have a flexible sole and ample cushioning. Do not choose the kind with very flared heels unless you run on extremely rough terrain because they can cause heel pain, tendonitis, or knee problems. People with flat feet or excessively high arches can sustain knee injuries. Leather or plastic inserts (orthodics) can dissipate the stress to the foot and help prevent these injuries. Without proper shoes, you might have foot, leg, knee or hip problems. If you do have problems, cut back drastically on the amount you exercise and find a good podiatrist who specializes in the problems of athletes. If possible, find one who engages in the same exercise you do.

Women who run a lot may be bothered with sweaty or bouncing breasts or irritated nipples. Many brands of sports bras are on the market today. Bras worn while running should be 55% to 100% cotton, a more absorbent fabric than synthetics. For maximum support, the back of the bra should be wide and fit low. Bras with padded seams are available that will eliminate the problem of sore nipples. Metal fasteners should be covered with fabric to prevent irritation.

Do not exercise in the morning without a light snack. If you do, you won't have sufficient carbohydrate available for the energy you need. This will cause an excessive liberation of stored fats leading to an increase in the amount of triglycerides in the blood. For people with a tendency toward hypoglycemia, eating something shortly before exercising is especially important because it avoids an episode of low blood sugar.

Do not exercise immediately after eating a heavy meal, especially one that is fatty. After such a meal, extra blood is diverted to the digestive tract and is not available to the heart and muscles which require more blood during exercise. If you have ingested a lot of fats, they will cause the red cells and platelets in the blood to stick together, blocking the capillaries and preventing the oxygen-carrying blood from reaching many muscle cells. When the skeletal muscles receive inadequate oxygen they will become fatigued. When the heart muscle does not obtain the oxygen it needs, the consequences are infinitely more serious.

Concentrated sweets, such as honey or candy bars, should be avoided immediately before and during strenuous exercise. They can cause the upper gastrointestinal tract to retain excessive amounts of water, and can lead to cramps, diarrhea, and to dehydration.

To increase circulation to the muscles, spend three to five minutes in pre-exercise and warm-up activities like jumping jacks or running in place. Do some exercises, like toe-touching, to stretch the muscles, tendons, and connective tissues. Just bend from the waist with your knees slightly bent and hang for thirty seconds without bouncing.

Bear in mind that running strengthens and tightens the muscles in the back of the leg but not the ones in the front. This could lead to foot, leg and knee problems. Therefore, you should do stretching exercises before and after jogging. The best exercise is keeping your feet flat on the ground while leaning forward with legs straight. Rest your hands against a stationary object about three or four feet away from you. Do this for several minutes. You will feel the pull in the calf muscles, especially if you have been a runner for some time. These precautions will lessen the chance of muscle tears or other injuries.

Do not overdress. It is better to be chilly when you start your run than to get overheated during it.

Immediately after strenuous exercise walk for a few minutes and cool down slowly. Blood has been brought to your muscles to supply oxygen and the other nutrients needed to meet the extra energy demands. Jogging, for instance, causes an increase of blood in the calf muscles. If you stop suddenly, without cooling down, this blood will cause congestion and a feeling of tightness from an accumulation of lactic acid. Lactic acid is formed from glucose in muscles during exercise. It contributes to fatigue and causes cramping. If you engage in new exercise without training, lactic acid saturation is reached sooner. Cooling down with light exercises flushes the accumulated blood and lactic acid from the muscles, decreasing the chances of discomfort afterwards.

Don't take a hot bath until at least thirty minutes after strenuous exercise. Exercise dilates the blood vessels supplying the muscles. Hot bathing will cause further dilation of these vessels and put a strain on the heart. Hot tubbing right after a work-out is especially dangerous. Soaking in warm water is a good way to relax tired muscles but wait thirty minutes to let your body functions come back to normal.

DIET AND EXERCISE

There is no special diet for people who exercise. The amount of protein we require is determined by how fast we are growing or how much we weigh and not by the degree of activity. Contrary to the myth, athletes need no more protein than sedentary people. A high protein diet can be dangerous since it contributes to dehydration. Remember that the waste products of protein metabolism are diluted with large amounts of water when they are eliminated. If a person who is not overweight exercises, he may have to consume more food—preferably carbohydrate—in order to meet his increased caloric needs.

When you exercise you don't need vitamin or mineral supplements. You will eat larger quantities of food to meet your increased caloric requirements. You will be less likely than other members of the population to be lacking in any nutrient. You must, however, eat enough to obtain as many calories as you expend.

When you exercise, you don't need more sodium (salt). In fact, excessive amounts of sodium can have an adverse effect on muscle efficiency. You are likely to need extra potassium and almost certain to need more water. You should drink adequate water or dilute fruit juices before, during and after exercising in order to prevent dehydration. Sweet drinks and caffeine beverages should be avoided since they can cause dehydration. Alcohol has an even greater dehydrating effect. Dehydration can be extremely dangerous when you are exercising, since water is needed for temperature control. It is also needed for energy production. Even mild exertion when you are dehydrated will cause the heart to beat faster. Performance is impaired when only 3% of the water in the body is lost; at 5% there will be signs of heat exhaustion; and at 7% hallucination will occur. Death will result if treatment is not immediate.

Excessive amounts of salt will cause sodium to accumulate in the fluid between the cells. This excess sodium pulls water from the cells causing them to become dehydrated. It also pulls water from the circulating blood resulting in a decrease in blood volume, which causes a person to perspire less profusely and can result in heat exhaustion.

It is *not* true that drinking water during exercise will cause cramps, but it is true that dehydration *can* have dire consequences. Dehydration is more apt to occur in people on a diet low in carbohydrates and high in protein and fat. With the exception of beans, which cause gas, only starchy foods should be eaten before vigorous exercise. Protein foods cause the formation of acids which cannot be excreted by the kidneys because of reduced blood flow to these organs during exercise. Fatty foods will not be readily broken down and are apt to cause indigestion.

Meat, other high protein foods and alcohol will make you hotter and should be avoided when exercising. In hot weather, it is best to exercise less strenuously. Otherwise there is danger of heat exhaustion. In hot weather a person perspires more profusely, increasing the risk of dehydration. Contrary to popular belief, if an athlete consumes a great deal of meat and other protein foods, he will not become stronger and more muscular, just fatter.

Although carbohydrates are the best source of fuel for athletes, carbohydrate loading is not a good idea. This practice involves eating in a special manner the week before an athletic event. For two and a half days a diet completely lacking in carbohydrates is followed. This depletes the muscles of glycogen, the stored carbohydrate. Then three days before an athletic event a large amount of carbohydrate is eaten to overload the stores of glycogen in the muscles. Some athletes use this technique before endurance type activities. It is not a good practice, especially in older people. Sometimes, it will cause so much glycogen and water to be deposited in the skeletal muscles that they feel stiff. And, more important, an overload of glycogen and water in the heart muscle can cause impaired cardiac function.

Many complicated processes of the body keep the individual cells healthy by supplying them with the nutrients they need. Ill health is often the result of cells getting too much food—especially certain kinds of food—and not getting enough oxygen. In the absence of sufficient oxygen, intermediate breakdown products of food will accumulate and can be converted to unhealthy or toxic substances.

Abstention from smoking and a regular program of aerobic exercise will result in an increase in the amount of oxygen received by the cells of the body. In addition to its aerobic effects, exercise has many other beneficial effects, both physical and emotional.

NUTRITION FOR A BETTER LIFE

I would like to summarize briefly the nutritional concepts of this book.

- We should eat many more carbohydrates, but they should be complex carbohydrates—starches and fiber.

- We should reduce the amount of simple carbohydrates (sugars) we eat—particularly extracted sugars.

- We should significantly cut down on the amount of fat in the diet—both saturated fat, as found in animal products, and unsaturated oils that have been extracted from plant foods.

- Cholesterol should be reduced in the diet by decreasing foods from animal sources.

- It is not necessary to consume much protein and we would be healthier if we consumed less.

- By eating more whole foods of plant origin, we will increase our consumption of fiber, the loss of which has been detrimental to our health.

- Our vitamin and mineral needs should be met by fresh fruits and vegetables, legumes and whole grains.

- We should avoid using salt at the table or in food preparation. The natural flavor of foods can be enhanced by using herbs and spices.

- If we do not exercise, we will be deficient in a most important nutrient—oxygen.

- Moderate drinking can cause liver damage and other problems. Occasional drinking will not have a significantly adverse effect on us if we do not have heart disease. It is not a good idea, however, to drink every day since it can be habit-forming or addictive. Exercise should be substituted for alcohol when trying to unwind.

- If you minimize extracted food fractions in your diet and eat mainly whole foods, you will greatly increase the quality of your life and possibly your longevity. I hope I have motivated you in this direction.

195

NOTES

All reference numbers refer to the bibliography, which follows.

CHAPTER 3 - How To Lose Weight   BIBLIOGRAPHY NUMBER

CHAPTER 4 - Carbohydrates   BIBLIOGRAPHY NUMBER

CHAPTER 10 - Alcohol   BIBLIOGRAPHY NUMBER

CHAPTER 11 - Beverages   BIBLIOGRAPHY NUMBER

CHAPTER 12 - Smoking   BIBLIOGRAPHY NUMBER

BIBLIOGRAPHY

1. Marx, J.L. 1977. Obesity—A Growing Problem. *Research News* December 2: 906-907.

2. Moss, N.H. and Mayer, J., eds. 1977. Food and Nutrition in Health and Disease. *Annals of the New York Academy of Sciences* 300: 1- 437.

3. Wurtman, R.J. and Wurtman, J.D. 1977. *Nutrition and the Brain.* Vol. 1. New York: Raven Press.

4. U.S. Senate Select Committee on Nutrition and Human Needs. 1977. *Dietary Goals for the United States.* U.S. Government Printing Office.

5. Rudzinska, M.A. 1951. The Influence of Amount of Food on the Reproduction Rate and Longevity of a Suctorian (Tokophrya infusionum). *Science* Vol. 113.

6. Ross, M.H. 1977. Dietary Behavior and Longevity. *Nutrition Reviews* 35: 257-265.

7. MacKeith, R.C. 1963. Is a Big Baby Healthy? *Proc. Nutr. Soc.* 22: 128-145.

8. Ross, M.H. 1961. Length of Life and Nutrition in the Rat. *Journal of Nutrition* 75: 197-210.

9. Dietary Preference, Growth, Aging and Lifespan. 1977. *Nutrition Reviews* 35 (2): 49-50.

10. Masoro, E.J., Bertrand, H. et al. 1979. Analysis and Exploration of Age-related Changes in Mammalian Structure and Function. *Federation Proc.* 38:1956-1961.

11. Porter, J.W.G. and Rolls, B.A. eds. 1973. *Proteins in Human Nutrition.* New York. Academic Press.

12. Sarles, H., Hauton, J., et al. 1977. Diet, Cholesterol, Gallstones and Composition of the Bile. *Digestive Diseases* 15(3): 251-260.

13. Schlenker, E.D., Feurig, J.S. et al. 1973. Nutrition and Health of Older People. *Am. J. Clin. Nutr.* 26:1111-1119.

14. Molina, R.M., Harper, A.B. et al. 1973. Age at Menarche in Athletes and Non-athletes. *Medicine and Science in Sports* 5(1): 11-13.

15. Frisch, R.E. and McArthur, J.W. 1974. Menstrual Cycles: Fatness as a Determinant of Minimum Weight for Height Necessary for Their Maintenance or Onset, *Science* 185: 949-951.

16. Frisch, R.E. 1974. A Method of Prediction of Age of Menarche from Height and Weight at Ages 9 through 13 Years. *Pediatrics* 53(3): 384-390.

17. Watt, B.K. and Merrill, A.L. 1963. *Composition of Foods, Agriculture Handbook No. 8.* U.S. Dept. of Agriculture.

18. Agriculture Research Service. 1976. *Composition of Foods—Dairy & Egg Products—Raw, Processed & Prepared—Agriculture Handbook No. 8-1.* U.S. Agriculture Research Service, Washington, D.C.

19. Settle, M.D. & Patterson, C.C. 1980. Lead in Albacore: Guide to Lead Pollution in America. *Science* 207: 1167-1176.

20. Expert Panel on Food, Safety and Nutrition. 1979. Dietary Fiber: A Scientific Status Summary by the IFT. *Food Technology* January, 35-39.

21. Food and Fiber. 1977. *Nutrition Reviews* 35(3): 52.

22. U.S. Food & Drug Administration. 1973. *Report on a Surveillance Program—Aflatoxin in Milk Products.* Bureau of Foods.

23. Edds, G.T. 1973. Acute Aflatoxosis: A Review. *JAVMA* 126: 304-309.

24. Carroll, K.K. 1978. Dietary Protein in Relation to Plasma Cholesterol Levels and Atherosclerosis. *Nutrition Reviews* 36(1): 1-5.

25. Effects of Drugs on the Fetus. 1973. *JAMA*, July 2:60.

26. Allport, S. 1980. DES Males' Reproductive Systems Get New Attention. *Medical Tribune* 21 (5): 19.

27. Gill, W.B., Schumacher, G.F.B. et al. 1979. Association of Diethylstilbestrol Exposure *in utero* with Cryptorchidism, Testicular Hypoplasia and Semen Abnormalities. *Journal of Urology* 122: 36-39.

28. Federal Register. August 3, 1979. 44 (151).

29. Confirmed by personal telephone communication with Constantine Zervos, Department of Health, Education and Welfare on March 25, 1980.

30. Comptroller General. April 17, 1979. *Problems in Preventing the Marketing of Raw Meat and Poultry Containing Potentially Harmful Residues.* Report to the Congress of the U.S.

31. Hall, R.H. 1974. *Food for Nought: The Decline in Nutrition.* San Francisco: Harper and Row.

32. Effect of Antibiotic Supplementation of Animal Feed on Human Intestinal Flora. 1977. *Nutrition Reviews* 35(4).

33. Gredon, J.F. 1979. Coffee, Tea and You. *The Sciences* 19(1): 6-11.

34. Commoner, B., Vithayathil, A.J. et al. 1978. Formation of Mutagens in Beef and Beef Extract During Cooking. *Science* 201: 913-916.

35. Peterson, D.W. 1951. Effect of Soybean Sterols in the Diet on Plasma and Liver Cholesterol in Chicks. *Proc. Soc. Exp. Biol. Med.* 78:143-147.

36. Pollack, O.J. 1953. Reduction of Blood Cholesterol in Man. *Circulation* 7:702-706.

37. Subbiah, M.T.R. 1973. Dietary Plant Sterols: Current Status in Human and Animal Sterol Metabolism. *Am. J. Clin. Nutr.* 26:219-225.

38. Plant Foods and Atherosclerosis. 1977. *Nutrition Reviews* 35(6):148-149.

39. Douglas, R. 1971. Letter. *Lancet* 2:7111.

40. Pfeiffer, C.C. 1975. *Mental and Elemental Nutrients.* New Canaan, Connecticut: Keats Publishing, Inc.

41. Wood, R., Chumbler, F. et al. 1977. Incorporation of Dietary *cis* and *trans* Isomers of Octadecenate in Lipid Classes of Liver and Hepatoma. *J. Biol. Chem.* 252(6):1965-1970.

42. Weiss, G. 1960. *Psychiatric Quarterly* 34:346-356.

43. Lovenberg, W. 1973. Some Vaso- and Psychoactive Substances in Food: Amines, Stimulants & Hallucinogens. In *Toxicants Occurring Naturally in Foods,* 2nd ed. National Academy of Sciences, Washington, D.C. p.181.

44. Dietz, W.H., Jr. and Stuart, M. 1976. Nutmeg and Prostaglandins. *The New England J. of Med.* 249(9).

45. Liener, I.E. 1969. *Toxic Constituents of Plant Foodstuffs.* San Francisco: Academic Press. p.413.

46. Schroeder, H.A. 1973. *The Trace Elements and Man.* Old Greenwich, Conn.: The Devin-Adair Company.

47. Too Much Sugar? 1978. *Consumer Reports.* March.

48. Hoover, R. and Strasser, H.S. *Progress Report to the Food and Drug Administration From the National Cancer Institute Concerning The National Bladder Cancer Study.* pp.2, 32-34.

49. Eastwood, M.A. 1977. Fibre and Enteropathic Circulation. *Nutrition Reviews.* 35:42.

50. Jain, R.C. 1977. Effect of Garlic on Serum Lipids, Coagulability and Fibrinolytic Activity of Blood (Letter). *Am. J. Clin. Nutr.* 30:1380-1381.

51. Bordia, A. & Bansol, H.C. 1973. Essential Oil of Garlic in Prevention of Atherosclerosis (letter). *Lancet* December 29:1491.

52. Van Elten, C.H. and Wolff, I.A. 1973. Natural Sulfur Compounds. In *Toxicants Occurring Naturally in Foods*, 2nd ed. Nat'l. Academy of Sciences, Washington, D.C. p.224.

53. Fujiwara, M. & Natata, T. 1967. Induction of Tumor Cells Treated With Extract of Garlic (Allium sativum) (letter) *Nature* 216:83-84.

54. Committee on Food Protection. Food & Nutrition Board. Nat'l Research Council. 1973. *Toxicants Occurring Naturally in Foods*. Washington, D.C.: Nat'l Acad. of Sciences.

55. Bordea, A., Bansol, H.C. et al. 1975. Effect of the Essential Oils of Garlic and Onion on Alimentary Hyperlipemia. *Atherosclerosis* Vol. 21.

56. Grande, F., Anderson, J. et al. 1965. Effect of Carbohydrates of Leguminous Seeds, Wheat & Potatoes on Serum Cholesterol Concentration in Man. *Nutrition* Vol. 86.

57. Borgstrom, G. 1968. *Principles of Food Science* Vol. 2. New York: The MacMillan Company.

58. McMillan, M. and Thompson, J.C. 1979. An Outbreak of Suspected Solanine Poisoning in Schoolboys: Examination of Criteria of Solanine Poisoning. *Quarterly J. of Med.* New Series 48(190):227-243.

59. Epstein, S.S. 1978..*The Politics of Cancer*. San Francisco: Sierra Club Books, pp.442-443.

60. Mayer, J., Roy, P. et al. 1956. Relation Between Caloric Intake, Body Weight and Physical Work: Studies in an Industrial Male Population in West Bengal. *Am. J. Clin. Nutr.* 4:169-175.

61. Haber, G.B., Heaton, K.W. et al. 1977. Depletion and Disruption of Dietary Fiber: Effect on Satiety, Plasma-Glucose, and Serum Insulin. *Lancet* Oct. 1.

62. Abrink, M.J. & Newman, T. 1979. Effect of High- and Low-Fiber Diets on Plasma Lipids and Insulin. *Am. J. Clin. Nutr.* 32(7):1486-1491.

63. Goette, D.K. and Odom, R.B. 1976. Alopecia in Crash Dieters. *J.A.M.A.* 235:2622-3.

64. Rickman, F., Mitchell, N. et al. 1974. Changes in Serum Cholesterol During the Stillman Diet. *JAMA* 228(1): 54–58.

65. Farquahar, J.W. 1978. *The American Way of Life Need Not Be Hazardous to Your Health*. Stanford, Ca.: Stanford Alumni Assoc.

66. Pectin. . .A Detoxifying Agent. 1963. *Citrus in Medicine* 2(1): 1–2.

67. Labuza, T.P. 1977. *Food and Your Well-Being*. Los Angeles: West Publishing Company.

68. Cohen, A.M. & Teitelbaum, A. 1964. Effect of Dietary Sucrose on Oral Glucose Tolerance and Insulin-like Activity. *Am. J. Physiol.* 206:105–8.

69. Bierman, E.L. 1979. Carbohydrates, Sucrose, and Human Disease. *Am. J. Clin. Nutr.* 32 (12): 2712–2722.

70. Cohen, A.M., Yudkin, J. 1967. The Effect of Dietary Sucrose Upon the Response to Sodium Tolbutamide in the Rat. *Biochemica et Biophysica Acta* 141:637.

71. Mayer, J. 1972. *Human Nutrition: Its Physiological, Medical and Social Aspects*. Springfield, Illinois: Charles C Thomas.

72. Ellestad, Sayed, J.J., & Haworth, J.C. 1977. Disaccharide Consumption and Malabsorption in Canadian Indians. *Amer. J. Clin. Nutr.* 30:698–703.

73. Cleave, T.L., Campbell, G.D. et al. 1969. *Diabetes, Coronary Thrombosis & the Saccharine Disease*. Bristol: John Wright.

74. Cohen, A.M. 1965. Fats and Carbohydrates as Factors in Atherosclerosis and Diabetes in Yemenite Jews. *American Heart Journal* 65(3).

75. Cohen, A.M., Bavly, S. et al. 1961. Change of Diet of Yemenite Jews in Relation to Diabetes and Ischemic Heart Disease. *The Lancet* 2:1399–1401.

76. Kuo, T., Feng, L. et al. 1967. Dietary Carbohydrates in Hyperlipemia (Hypertriglyceridemia); Hepatitus & Adipose Tissue Lipogenic Activities. *Amer. J. Clin. Nutr.* 20:116–125

77. Yudkin, J. and Roddy, J. 1964. Levels of Dietary Sucrose in Patients With Occlusive Atherosclerotic Disease. *The Lancet* 2:6–8.

78. Yudkin, J. & Krauss, R. 1967. Dietary Starch, Dietary Sucrose & Hepatic Pyruvate Kinase in Rats. *Nature* 215:75.

79. Bruckerdorfer, K.R., Khan, I.H. et al. 1971. Dietary Carbohydrate & Fatty Acid Synthetase Activity in Rat Liver & Adipose Tissue. *Biochemical Journal 123:7.*

80. *Abrens, R.A., Demuth, P. et al. 1980. Moderate Sucrose Ingestion and Blood Pressure in the Rat. J. Nutr.* 110 (in press).

81. Tappel, A.L. 1968. Will Antioxidant Nutrients Slow Aging Processes? *Geriatrics*, Oct.

82. Bjorksten, J. 1968. The Crosslinkage Theory of Aging. *Journal of the American Geriatrics* 16(4).

83. Ritchie, J.H., Fish, M.B. et al. 1970. Edema and Hemolytic Anemia in Premature Infants: A Vitamin E Deficiency Syndrome. *New Eng. Journal of Medicine* 279:1185–1968.

84. Holman, R. 1979. The Deficiency of Essential Fatty Acids. In *Polyunsaturated Fatty Acids*, ed. H. Kunan Wolf & R.T. Holman, Champaign, Illinois: American Oil Chemists' Society. p. 168.

85. Hughes, L. *Heartscan, The Handbook*. Santa Cruz, California: Heartscan, Inc.

86. Dock, W. 1958. Research in Atherosclerosis——The First Fifty Years. *Ann. Internal Med.* 49:699.

87. Connor, W.E. and Connor S.L. 1972. The Key Role of Nutritional Factors in the Prevention of Coronary Heart Disease. *Prev. Med.* 1:49

88. Connor, W.E., Cerquiera, M.T. et al. 1978. The Plasma Lipids, Lipoproteins, and the Diet of the Tarahumara Indians of Mexico. *Amer. J. Clin. Nutr.* 31(7).

89. Leonard, J.N., Hofer, J.L. et al. 1974. *Live Longer Now.* New York: Grosset and Dunlap. p. 30–35.

90. U.S. Dept. of Health, Education and Welfare. 1979. *Healthy People: The Surgeon General's Report on Health Promotion and Disease Prevention.*

92. Spritz, N., Ahrens, E.H., Jr. et al. 1965. Sterol Balance in Man as Plasma Cholesterol Concentrations are Altered by Exchange of Dietary Fats. *J. Clin. Invest.* 44(9):1482.

93. Glueck, C.J. 1979. Dietary Fat and Atherosclerosis. *A. J. Clin. Nutr. 32(12):2703–2711.*

94. *Harman, D. 1968. Free Radical Theory of Aging: Effect of Free Radical Inhibitors on the Mortality Rate of Male LAF Mice. Gerontology 23:476.*

95. Carpenter, D.G. and Loynd, J.A. 1968. An Integrated Theory of Aging. *Journal of the American Geriatrics Society*, Vol. XVI, No. 12.

96. Roen, P.B. 1978. The Evening Meal and Atherosclerosis. *J. Am. Geriatrics Society* 26(6):284–5.

97. Enos, W.F., Holmes, R.H. et al. 1953. Coronary Disease Among U.S. Soldiers Killed in Action in Korea. *J.A.M.A.* 152:1090.

98. Kannel, W.B., Castelli, W.P. et al. 1967. The Coronary Profile: Twelve Year Follow-Up in the Framingham Study. *J. Occup. Med.* 9:611.

99. Chapman, J.M. and Massey, F., Jr. 1964. The Interrelationship of Serum Cholesterol, Hypertension, Body Weight, and Risk of Coronary Disease. *J. Chron. Dis.* 17:933.

100. Kannel, W.B., Castelli, W.P. et al. 1971. Serum Cholesterol Lipoproteins and the Risk of Coronary Heart Disease. The Framingham Study. *Ann. Int. Med.* 74:1-12.

101. Connor, W.E., Hodges, R.E. et al. 1961. The Serum Lipids in Men Receiving High Cholesterol and Cholesterol-Free Diets. *J. Clin. Invest.* 40:894.

102. Hegsted, D.M., McGandy, R.B. et al. 1965. Quantitative Effects of Dietary Fat on Serum Cholesterol in Man. *Am. J. Clin. Nutr.* 17:281-295.

103. Beveridge, J.M.R., Connell, W.F. et al. 1959. Dietary Cholesterol and Plasma Cholesterol Levels in Man. *Canad. J. Biochem. Physiol.* 37:575-582.

104. Connor, W.E., Hodges, R.E. et al. 1961. The Serum Lipids in Men Receiving High Cholesterol and Cholesterol-Free Diets. *J. Clin. Invest.* 40:894-901.

105. Stammler, J. 1978. Dietary and Serum Lipids in the Multifactorial Etiology of Atherosclerosis. *Arch Surg.* 113:21-25.

106. Mattson, F.H., Erickson, B.A. et al. 1972. Effect of Dietary Cholesterol on Serum Cholesterol in Man. *Am. J. Clin. Nutr.* 25:589-594.

107. Connor, W.E. 1961. Dietary Cholesterol and the Pathogenesis of Atherosclerosis. *Geriatrics* 16:407-415.

108. Erickson, B.A., Coots, R.H. et al. 1964. The Effect of Partial Hydrogenation of Polyunsaturated to Saturated Fatty Acids and of Dietary Cholesterol upon Plasma Lipids in Man. *J. Clin. Invest.* 43:2017.

109. Borgstrom, B. 1969. Quantification of Cholesterol Absorption in Man by Fecal Analysis after the Feeding of a Single Isotope-labeled Meal. *J. Lip. Res.* 10:331.

110. McGill, H.C., Jr., ed. 1968. *Geographic Pathology of Atherosclerosis.* Baltimore, Maryland: Williams & Wilkins Co.

111. Keys, A. 1970. Coronary Heart Disease in Seven Countries. *Circulation* 41 (Supp. 1):1-211.

112. Keys, A., Aravanis, C. et al. 1966. Epidemiological Studies Related to Coronary Heart Disease: Characteristics of Men Aged 40-59 in Seven Countries. *Acta Med Scand.* 460:1-392.

113. National Academy of Sciences. 1974. *Water Deprivation and Performance of Athletes.* May.

114. Hankin, J., Reed, D. et al. 1970. Dietary and Disease Patterns Among Micronesians. *Amer. J. Clin Nutr.* 23(2):346-351.

115. Krueger, D.E. and Moriyama, I.M. 1967. Mortality of the Foreign Born. *Amer. J. Pub. Health* 57:496.

116. Nes, W.R. and McKean, M.L. 1977. *Biochemistry of Steroids and Other Isopentenoids.* Baltimore, Maryland: University Park Press.

117. McGill, H.C. 1979. The Relationship of Dietary Cholesterol Concentration and Atherosclerosis in Man. *Am. J. Clin. Nutr.* 32:2664-2702.

118. Miller, G.J. and Miller N.E. 1975. Plasma-High-Density-Lipoprotein Concentrations and Development of Ischaemic Heart Disease. *Lancet* 1:16-19.

119. Rhoads, G.G., Gulbrandsen, C.L. & Kagan, A. 1976. Serum Lipoproteins and Coronary Heart Disease in a Population Study of Hawaii Japanese Men. *N. Eng. J. of Med.* 294:293-298.

120. .Trowell, H. Jan 20, 1978. Lecture delivered at the Second Annual Longeveity Research Institute Conference. Santa Barbara, Calilfornia.

121. Lea, A.J. 1966. Dietary Factors Associated with Death-Rates from Certain Neoplasms in Man. *Lancet* 2:332-333.

122. Wynder, E. Jan. 11, 1979. *Nutritional Carcinogenesis.* Lecture delivered at the Third Annual Educational Conference at the Longevity Research Institute. Santa Monica, California.

123. Carroll, K.K. & Hopkins, G.J. 1979. Dietary Polyunsaturated Fat versus Saturated Fat in Relation to Mammary Carcinogenesis. *Lipis* 14(2):155-158.

124. Gammal, E.B., Carroll, K.K., and Plunkett, E.R. 1967. Effects of Dietary Fat on Mammary Carcinogenesis by 7, 12-Dimethylbenz(a)Anthracene in Rats. *Cancer Res.* 27:1737.

125. Denham, H. 1969. Prolongation of Life: Role of Free Radical Reactions in Aging. *J. Am. Geriatr. Soc.* 17:721.

126. Hill, M.J. 1971. Bacteria and Aetiology of Cancer of the Large Bowel. *Lancet* 1:95-100.

127. Hill, M.J. 1974. Steroid Nuclear Dehydration and Colon Cancer. *Am. J. Clin. Nutr.* 27:1475-1480.

128. Wynder, E.L. 1977. Nutritional Carcinogenesis. In *Food and Nutrition in Health and Disease*, eds N.H. Moss and J. Mayer, pp. 360-378.

129. Haenzel, W. and Kurehara, M. 1973. Studies of Japanese Migrants: I. Mortality from Cancer and Other Diseases Among Japanese in the U.S. *Nat'l. Cancer Inst.* 51:1765-1779.

130. Wynder, E., Kajitani, T. et al. Environmental Factors of Cancer of the Colon and Rectum, II. Japanese Epidemiological Data. *Cancer* 23:1210.

131. Pearce, M.L. and Dayton, S. 1971. Incidence of Cancer in Men on a Diet High in Polyunsataturated Fat. *Lancet* 1:464-467.

132. Finegold, S.M., Attebury, H.R., & Sutter, V.L. 1974. Effect of Diet on Human Fecal Flora: Comparison of Japanese & American Diets. *Amer. J. Clin. Nutr.* 27:1456.

133. Hill, M.J. Goddard, P. et al. 1971. Gut Bacteria and Aetiology of Cancer of the Breast. *Lancet* II:472.

134. Stare, J. & McWilliams, M. 1977. *Living Nutrition.* Santa Barbara, Ca.: John Wiley & Sons.

135. MacKay, E.M., Barnes, R.H. et al. 1940. Ketogenic Activity of Acetic Acid. *J. Biol. Chem.* 135:157.

136. Jowsey, J. 1971. *Metabolic Diseases of Bone.* W.B. Saunders Co. pp. 248-303.

137. Armenian, H.K., Lilienfeld, A.M. et al. 1974. Relation Between Benign Prostatic Hyperplasia and Cancer of the Prostate. *Lancet* 2:115-117.

138. Hill, P., Wynder, E.L. et al. 1979. Diet and Urinary Steroids in Black and White North American Men and Black South African Men. *Cancer Research* 39:5101-5105.

139. Melchior, G.W., Lofland, H.B.. et al. 1974. Influence of Dietary Fat on Cholelithiasis in Squirrel Monkeys. *Fed. Proc.* 33:626.

140. Walford, R.L. 1962. Autoimmunity and Aging. *J. Gerontol.* 2:281-285.

141. Stroud, M. 1974. A Family of Protein-Cutting Proteins. *Scientific American* July.

142. Roberts, S. & Caserio, M.C. 1971. *Organic Chemistry: Methane to Macromolecules.* Menlo Park, Ca.: W.A. Benjamin, Inc.

143. U.S. Federal Trade Commission. Jan 15, 1979. *Advertising and Labeling of Protein Supplements.* pp.121-127.

144. United States of America Before Federal Trade Commission. Report of the Presiding Officer (Christopher W. Keller) 1978. *Proposed Trade Regulation Rule Regarding Advertising & Labeling of Protein Supplements.*

145. *McClaren, D.S. 1974. Dietary Protein in Medical Practice. The Practitioner* 212:441.

146. U.S. Federal Trade Comm. Jan 15, 1979. *Advertising and Labeling of Protein Supplements.* p.115.

147. Sukhatme, P.V. & Margen, S. 1978. Models for Protein Deficiency. *Am. J. Clin. Nutr.* 31:1237-1256.

148. F.A.O./W.H.O. Expert Committee. 1973. *Energy and Protein Requirements.* FAO Nutritional Meeting, Report Serial No. 52. WHO Technical Report Serial No. 522.

149. Lamb, L.E. *Metabolics: Putting Your Food Energy to Work.* New York: Harper & Row.

150. U.S. Federal Trade Comm. Jan 15, 1979. *Advertising and Labeling of Protein Supplements.* pp. 27-35.

151. Ibid., pp. 116-121.

152. Palombo, J.D. & Blackburn, G.L. 1980. Human Protein Requirements. *Contemporary Nutrition* 5(1).

153. Abernathy, R.P., Ritchey, S.J. et al. 1972. Lack of Response to Amino Acid Supplements by Preadolescent Girls. *Amer. J. Clin Nutr.* 25:980-982.

154. Burkett, D.P. and Trowell, H.C., eds. 1975. *Refined Carbohydrate Foods and Disease: Some Implications of Dietary Fibre.* New York: Academic Press.

155. Jowsey, J. 1976. Prevention and Treatment of Osteoporosis. In *Nutrition and Aging,* ed. M. Winick, New York: John Wiley & Sons. pp. 131-144.

156. Ellis, F.R. Holesh, S. et al. 1972. Incidence of Osteoporosis in Vegetarians and Omnivores. *Amer. J. Clin Nutr.* 25:555-8.

157. U.S. Federal Trade Comm. Jan. 15, 1979. *Advertising and Labeling of Protein Supplements.* pp. 232-244.

158. Ibid., pp. 180-207.

159. Ibid., pp. 167-180.

160. Gainer, J.L. and Chisolm, G.M. III, 1974. Oxygen Diffusion and Atherosclerosis. *Atherosclerosis* 19:135-138.

161. Nitrogen Intake and Tumorigenesis in Rats. 1977. *Nutrition Reviews* 35(4).

162. Van Soest, P.J. and Robertson, J.B. 1977. What is Fibre and Fibre in Food? *Nutrition Reviews* 35:15.

163. Dietary Fiber as a Binder of Bile Salts. 1977. *Nutrition Reviews* 35(7):183-185.

164. Trowell, H. 1976. Definition of Dietary Fiber and Hypotheses That it is a Protective Factor in Certain Diseases. *Am. J. Clin. Nutr.* 29:417-427.

165. Trowell, H. 1977. Food and Dietary Fibre. *Nutrition Reviews* 35:6-7.

166. *Nutrition Reviews.* 1977. 35:55-70.

167. The Role of Fiber in the Diet. 1975. *Dairy Council Digest* 46(1):2.

168. Burkitt, D. & Meisner, P. 1979. How to Manage Constipation With High-fiber Diet. *Geriatrics* Feb.:33-40.

169. *Harrison's Principles of Internal Medicine, 6th ed.* McGraw-Hill Book Company. 1970.

170. Burkitt, D.P. 1971. Diverticular Disease of the Colon; A Deficiency Disease of Western Civilization. *British Medical Journal* 2:450-454.

171. Latto, C., Wilkenson, R.W. et al. 1973. Diverticular Disease and Varicose Veins. *Lancet* May 19:1089-1090.

172. Goldstein, F. 1972. Diet and Colonic Disease. *Journal of the American Dietetic Association* 60:499-503.

173. Fleiszer, D., MacFarlane, J. et al. 1978. Protective Effect of Dietary Fibre Against Chemically Induced Bowel Tumours in Rats. *Lancet* Sept. 19.

174. Burkitt, D. 1979. Eat Right—To Stay Healthy and Enjoy Life More. New York: Arco Publishing, Inc.

175. Short, A.R. 1920. The Causation of Appendicitis. *British Journal of Surgery* 8:171-186.

176. Bennet, P.H., Burch, T.A. et al. 1971. Diabetes Mellitus in American (Pima) Indians. *Lancet* 2:125-128.

177. Vinik, A.I., Smith, C. et al. Effect of Dietary Fiber on Serum Glucose and Insulin Responses With and Without Autonomic Neuropathy and in Healthy Controls. *Diabetes* 82:384-385.

178. Hall, S.E.H., Bolton, T.M. et al. 1979. Can Bran Increase Insulin Sensitivity? *Diabetes* 82:384-385.

179. Cummings, J.H. 1978. Nutritional Implications of Dietary Fiber. *Am J. Clin Nutr.* Oct. 31:521-529.

180. Brodribb, A.J.M. and Humphreys, D.M. 1976. Diverticular Disease: Three Elements, Part I—Relation to Other Disorders and Fiber Intake. *British Medical Journal* Feb. 21:424-425.

181. Morris, J.N., Marr, J.W. et al. 1977. Diet and Heart: A Postscript. *British Medical Journal* 2:1307-1314.

182. Brown, J., Bourke, G.J. et al. Nutritional and Epidemiologic Factors Related to Heart Disease. *World Review of Nutrition and Dietetics* 12:1-42.

183. Capron, J., Dumont, M. et al. 1978. Evidence For an Association Between Cholelithiasis and Hiatus Hernia. *Lancet* II:8085.

184. Takton, M.D. 1968. *The Great Vitamin Hoax.* New York: The Macmillan. Co.

185. Hayes, K.C. and Hegsted, D.M. 1973. Toxicants of the Vitamins. In: *Toxicants Occurring Naturally in Foods.* National Academy of Sciences.

186. McCormick, D.B. 1979. Dangers of Overdose of Water-soluble Vitamins. *Nutrition and the M.D.* 5(10):1-2.

187. Robinson, R.A. 1966. *The Vitamin Co-Factors of Enzyme Systems.* New York: Pergamon Press.

188. Goodhart, R.S. and Shils, M.E. 1973. *Modern Nutrition in Health and Disease.* 5th ed. Philadelphia: Lea and Febiger.

189. National Academy of Sciences. 1974. *Recommended Daily Dietary Allowances.*

190. Sebrell, W.H., Jr., and Harris, R.S. 1971. *The Vitamins: Chemistry, Physiology, Pathology, Methods.* New York: Academic Press, pp.386-387.

191. Herbert, V. 1979. Pangamic Acid ("Vitamin B_{15}"). *Am. J. Clin. Nutr.* 32:1534-1540.

192. Von Haller, A. 1962. *The Vitamin Hunters.* New York: Chilton Company.

193. Fennema, O. 1977. Loss of Vitamins in Fresh and Frozen Foods. *Food Technology* 31(12).

194. Lewin, S. 1976. *Vitamin C: Its Molecular Biology and Medical Potential.* San Francisco: Academic Press.

195. Marks, J. 1968. *The Vitamins in Health and Disease: A Modern Reappraisal.* Boston, Mass.: Little, Brown and Company.

196. Vitamin C and Phagocyte Function. 1978. *Nutrition Reviews* 36(6):183-185.

197. Collier, P. 1978. The Old Man and the C. *New West*, p.21-25, April.

198. *Nutrition and the M.D.* 1979. 5(10):1-2.

199. National Nutrition Consortium, Inc. 1978. *Vitamin-Mineral Safety, Toxicity, and Misuse.* Chicago: The American Dietetic Association.

200. Levy. J.B. and Bach-y-Rita, P. 1976. *Vitamins: Their Use and Abuse.* New York: Liveright.

201. Briggs, M.H., Webb-Garcia, P. et al. 1973. Urinary Oxalate and Vitamin C Supplements (letter). *Lancet.* July 29:201.

202. Herbert, V. and Jacob, E. 1974. Destruction of Vitamin B_{12} by Ascorbic Acid. *JAMA* 230(2):241-242.

203. Klevay, L.M. 1978. Hypercholesterolemia Due to Ascorbic Acid. *Proc. Soc. Exper. Biol. Med.* 151:579-582.

204. Greenberg, R., Cornbleet, T. et al. 1959. Accumulation and Excretion of Vitamin A-Like Flourescent Material By Sebaceous Glands after the Oral Administration of Various Carotenoids. *J. Invest Dermatol.* 32:599-604.

205. Josephs, H. 1944. Hypervitaminosis A and Carotenemia. *Am. J. Dis. Child.* 67:33-43.

206. Kordylas, J. 1972. Vitamin-A and Fat Combination in Cholesterol Biosynthesis and Atherosclerosis (letter). *Lancet* Sep. 16, p.606.

207. Kirschmann, J. 1975. *Nutrition Almanac.* New York: McGraw-Hill Book Co.

208. Wurtman, R. 1975. The Effects of Light on the Human Body. *Scientific American* July, pp.69-77.

209. Ehrlich, P., Tarver, H. et al. 1972. Inhibitory Effects of Vitamin E on Collagen Synthesis and Wound Repair. *Ann. Surg.* 175:235-240.

210. Vitamin E. 1977. *Nutrition Reviews.* 35(2):57-62.

211. Tappel, A.L. 1973. Vitamin E. *Nutrition Today.* July/Aug. p.4.

212. Chow, C.K. and Tappel, A.K. 1972. An Enzymatic Protective Mechanism Against Lipid Peroxidation Damage to Lungs of Exposed Rat. *Lipids* 7:518.

213. Chow, C.K. and Kaneko, J.J. 1979. Influence of Dietary Vitamin E on the Red Cells of Ozone-exposed Rats. *Environmental Research.* 19:45-55.

214. Marusiche, W.L., De Ritter, E. et al. 1975. Effect of Supplemental Vitamin E in Control of Rancidity in Poultry Meat. *Poultry Science* 54:831-844.

215. Vitamin E: *Questions and Answers.* 1979. Minneapolis: Henkel Corp.

216. Tsai, A.C., Kelley, J.J. et al. 1978. Study of the Effect of Megavitamin E Supplementation in Man. *Am. J. Clin. Nutr.* 31:831-837.

217. Ayers, S., Jr. 1973. Natural vs. Synthetic Vitamins. *JAMA* 225(9):1124.

218. Butterworth, C.E., Jr. 1974. The Skeleton in the Hospital Closet. *Nutrition Today* March/April. pp.4-8.

219. The National Research Council. 1978, *Geochemistry and the Environment.*

220. Oxalates. 1979. *Nutrition and the M.D.* 5(9):3.

221. Mellanby, Sir Edward. 1950. *A Story of Nutritional Research: The Effect of Some Dietary Factors on Bones and the Nervous System.* Baltimore: The Willilams & Wilkens Company.

222. Norman, A.W. and Henry, H.L. 1979. Vitamin D to 1,25-dihydroxycholecalciferol: Evolution of a Steroid Hormone. *Trends in Biochemical Sciences* 4(1):14-18.

223. Bassett, C.A. 1971. Effect of Force on Skeletal Tissue. In *Physiological Basis of Rehabilitation Medicine,* eds. J.A. Downey and R.C. Darling, p.312. W.B. Saunders Company.

224. Wachman, A. and Bernstein, D.S. 1968. Diet and Osteoporosis. *The Lancet*: May 4.

225. Solomon, L. 1968. Osteoporosis and Fracture of the Femoral Neck in the South African Bantu. *Journal of Bone and Joint Surgery* 50B(1):2-13.

226. Agricultural Research Service. U.S. Dept. of Agriculture. 1975. *Nutritive Values of American Foods in Common Units, Agriculture Handbook, No. 456.*

227. Belanger, L.F. 1972. Calcium-Phosphorus Balance and Periodontal Disease. In *Mineral Nutrition Today, Proceedings of the Miles Symposium.* pp.35-45. Nutrition Society of Canada.

228. Anderson. T.W., Neri, L.C. et al. 1975. Ischemic Heart Disease, Water Hardness and Myocardial Magnesium. *Canadian Mediacl Association Journal* 13:199-203.

229. Johnson, C.J., Peterson, D.R. et al. 1979. Myocardial Tissue Concentration of Magnesium and Potassium in Men Dying Suddenly from Ischemic Heart Disease. *Am. J. Clin. Nutr.* 32:967-970.

230. Mount, J.L. 1975. *The Food and Health of Western Man*. London: Charles Knight & Company Limited.

231. United States Department of Agriculture. *Nutrition and Your Health: Dietary Guide for Americans* Food & Garden Bulletin No. 228.

232. Tobian, L. 1979. The Relationship of Salt to Hypertension. *Am. J. Clin Nutr.* 32:2739-2748.

233. Cook, J.D. and Finch, C.A. 1972. Iron Deficiency in Man. In *Mineral Nutrition Today. Proceedings of the Miles Symposium*. Nutrition Society of Canada.

234. Brewer, G.J. and Prasad, A.S., eds. 1977. *Zinc Metabolism: Current Aspects in Health and Disease*. New York: Alan R. Liss, Inc.

235. Hall "O" Ok, T. and Hedelin, H. 1971. Zinc Metabolism and Surgical Trauma. *British Journal of Surgery* 64(4):271-3.

236. Orris, L., Shalita, A.R. et al. 1978. Oral Zinc Therapy of Acne. *Arch. Dermatol.* 114(7):1018-20.

237. Dronfield, M.W., Malone, J.D. et al. 1977. Zinc in Ulcerative Colitis: A Therapeutic Trial and Report on Plasma Levels. *Gut* 18(1):33-6.

238. Weisman, K. 1978. What Is the Use of Zinc for Wound Healing? *International Journal of Dermatology* 17:568-570.

239. Holden, J.M., Wolf, W.R. et al. 1979. Zinc and Copper in Self-selected Diets. *J. of the American Dietetic Assoc.* 75(1):23-8.

240. Gregor, J.L., Higgins, M.M. et al. 1978. Nutritional Status of Adolescent Girls in Regard to Zinc, Copper and Iron. *Am. J. Clin. Nutr.* 31(2):269-75.

241. Klevay, L.M. 1975. Coronary Heart Disease: The Zinc/Copper Hypothesis. *Am J. Clin. Nutr.* 28:764-774.

242. Wallenius, K., Mather, A. et al. 1979. Effects of Different Levels of Dietary Zinc on Development of Chemically Induced Oral Cancer in Rats. *Int. Journal Oral Surg.* 8(1):56-62.

243. Oberleas, D., Caldwell, D. et al. 1972. Trace Elements and Behavior. In *Neurobiology of the Trace Minerals Zinc and Copper*. ed. C. Pfeiffer. New York: Academic Press.

244. Pfeiffer, C.C. and Venelin, I. 1972. A Study of Zinc Deficiency and Copper Excess in the Schizophrenias. In *Neurobiology of the Trace Metals Zinc and Copper*. ed. C.C. Pfeiffer. New York: Academic Press. pp.141-165.

245. National Academy of Sciences. 1976. *Selenium and Human Health*. September.

246. Selenium and Human Health. 1976. *Nutrition Reviews* 34(11):347-348.

247. Morris, V.C. and Levander, O.A. 1970. Selenium Content of Foods. *Nutrition* 100:1383-1388.

248. National Academy of Sciences. 1971. *Flourides*.

249. Bendz, G. and Linquist, I., eds. 1978. *Biochemistry of Silicon and Related Problems*. New York: Plenum Press.

250. Prasad, A.S., ed. 1976. *Trace Elements in Human Nutrition Vol II*. New York: Academic Press.

251. Settle, D.M. and Patterson, C.C. 1980. Lead in Albacore: Guide to Lead Pollution in Americans. *Science* 207:1167-1176.

252. National Academy of Sciences. 1972. *Lead*.

253. U.S. Department of Health, Education and Welfare. 1971. *Lead in Food: Advance Notice of Proposed Rulemaking*. Federal Register Vol. 44, No. 171. p.51233-51242.

254. Lehmann, P. 1979. *Food and Drug Interactions*. HEW Publication No. (FDA) 78-3070.

255. Forney, R.B. and Hughes, F.W. 1968. *Combined Effect of Alcohol and Other Drugs*. Springfield, Ill.: Charles C Thomas.

256. Burton, B.T. 1976. *Human Nutrition, 3rd ed.* McGraw-Hill Book Co. pp.416-419.

257. Mutch, P. 1979. In Animals, the Equivalent of 9 Cups of Coffee a Day Whets Alcohol Urge. *Medical Tribune* 20(35):3.

258. Lieber, C.S. 1967. Alcoholic Fatty Liver, Hyperlipemia and Hyperuricemia. In *Biochemical Factors in Alcoholism*. ed. R.P. Maickel. New York: Pergamon Press.

259. Maling, H.M., Highman, B. et al. 1967. Blood Cholesterol Levels, Triglyceride Fatty Livers and Pathologic Changes in Rats After Single Large Doses of Alcohol. In *Biochemical Factors in Alcoholism*. ed. R.P. Maickel. New York: Pergamon Press.

260. U.S. Dept. of Health, Education and Welfare. 1978. *Alcohol and Health*.

261. Patek, A.J., Jr. 1979. Alcohol, Malnutrition and Alcoholic Cirrhosis. *Am. J. Clin. Nutr.* 32:1304-1312.

262. Spritz, N. 1979. Review of the Evidence Linking Alcohol Consumption With Liver Disease and Atherosclerotic Disease. *Am. J. Clin. Nutr.* 32(12):2734-2738.

263. Gould, L., Zahir, M. et at. 1971. Cardiac Effects of a Cocktail. *JAMA* 218(12):1799.

264. Van Thiel, D.H. and Lester, R. 1967. Alcoholism: Its Effect on Hypothalmic Pituitary Gonad Function. *Gastroenterology* 71:318-327.

265. Stephenson, P.E. 1977. Physiologic and Psychotropic Effects of Caffeine on Man. *J. Am. Diet. Assoc.* 71(3):240-7.

266. Bunker, M.L. and McWilliams, M. 1979. Caffeine Content of Common Beverages. *J. Am. Diet. Assoc.* 74(1):28-32.

267. Robertson, D., Frohlich, J.C. et al. 1978. Effects of Caffeine on Plasma Renin Activity, Catecholamines and Blood Pressure. *New England Journal of Medicine* 298:181-186.

268. Palm, P.E., Arnold, E.P. et al. 1978. Evaluation of the Teratogenic Potential of Fresh-brewed Coffee and Caffeine in the Rat. *Toxicology and Applied Pharmacology* 44:1-16.

269. Ax, R.L., Collier, R.J. et al. 1976. Effects of Dietary Caffeine on the Testes of the Domestic Fowl *Gallus domesticans. J. Reprod. Fert.* 47:235-238.

270. Thayer, P. and Kensler, C.J. 1973. Genetic Tests in Mice of Caffeine Alone and in Combination with Mutagens. *Toxicol. Appl. Pharm.* 25:157-168.

271. Friedman, L., Weinberger, M. et al. 1975. Testicular Atrophy and Aspermatogenesis in Rats Fed Caffeine or Theobromine in the Presence or Absence of Sodium Nitrite. *Fed. Proc.* 34:228.

272. Minton, J.P., Foecking, M.K. et al. 1979. Response of Fibrocystic Disease to Caffeine Withdrawal and Correlation of Cyclic Nucleotides with Breast Disease. *Am. J. Clin. Nutr.* 135(1):157-8.

273. Minton, J.P., Foecking, M.K. et al. 1979. Caffeine, Cyclic Nucleotides, and Breast Disease. *Surgery* 86(1):105-9.

274. Lutz, E.G. 1978. Restless Legs, Anxiety and Caffeinism. *J. Clin. Psychiatry* 39(9):693-8.

275. Challis, B.C. and Bartlett, C.D. 1975. Possible Carcinogenic Effects of Coffee Constituents. *Nature* 254:532-533.

276. Kalsner, S. 1977. A Coronary Vasoconstrictor is Present in Regular and "Decaffeinated" Forms of Both Percolated and Instant Coffee. *Life Sci.* 20(10):1689-96.

277. Groisser, D.S. 1978. A Study of Caffeine in Tea. *Am. J. Clin. Nutr.* 31(10):1727-31.

278. Kositawattanakul, T., Tosukhowong, P. et al. 1977. Chemical Interactions Between Thiamin and Tannic Acid. *Am. J. Clin. Nutr.* 30(10):1686-91.

279. De Alacron, P.A., Donovan, M. 1979. Iron Absorption in the Thalassemia Syndrome and its Inhibition by Tea. *New England Journal of Medicine* 300:5-8.

280. Morton, Julia F. to Bronfen. 18 March 1980.

281. Vimokesant, S.L. and Miller, D.M. 1975. Effects of Betel Nut and Fermented Fish on the Thiamin Status of Northeastern Thais. *Am. J. Clin. Nutr.* 28:1458-1463.

282. Morton, J.F. 1979. (letter). *Science* June 1, p. 909.

283. Tsushida, T. and Takeo, T. 1977. Zinc, Copper, Lead and Cadmium Contents in Green Tea. *J. Sci. Food Agric.* 28(3):255-8.

284. Siegal, R.K. 1979. Ginseng Abuse Syndrome. *JAMA* 241(15):1614-15.

285. Toxic Reactions to Plant Products Sold in Health Food Stores. 1979. *The Medical Letter* 21:29-31.

286. Morton, J.F. 1974. Is There a Safer Tea? Presented at the American Society of Pharmacognosy and Academy of Pharmaceutical Sciences Section on Pharmacognosy and Natural Products Joint Meeting, University of Illinois, Aug. 6.

287. Econews—Newsletter of the North Coast Environmental Center 9(12):16, 1979.

288. MacDonald, J. and Margen, S. 1979. Wine Versus Ethanol in Human Nutrition. *Am. J. Clin. Nutr.* 32(4):823-833.

289. Berland, T. 1972. Wine Served in Hospitals. *The Cornell Hotel and Restaurant Administration Quarterly* 13:63.

290. Trethewie, E.R. 1979. Wines and Headaches (letter). *Med. J. of Australia* 1(3):94.

291. Bruno, P., Caselli, M. et al. 1978. Simultaneous Determination of Copper, Lead and Zinc in Wine by Differential-pulse Polarography. *Analyst* 103:687-71.

292. Wai, C.M., Knowles, C.R. et al. 1979. Lead Caps on Wine Bottles and Their Potential Problems. *Bull. Environm. Contam. Toxicol.* 21:4-6.

293. Lucia, S.P. 1971. *Wine and Your Well-Being.* New York: Popular Library, p. 46.

294. Keating, J.P., Lell, M.E. et al. 1973. Infantile Methemglobinemia Caused by Carrot Juice. *The New England Journal of Medicine* 228(16):824-826.

295. The National Research Council. 1977. *Drinking Water and Health.*

296. Cooper, R.C., Kanarek, M. et al. 1978. *Asbestos in Domestic Water Supplies in Five California Counties.* Division of Environmental Health Sciences, School of Public Health, Univ. of California, Berkeley, p.77.

297. Dawson, E.B., Frey, M.J. et al. 1978. Relationship of Metal Metabolism to Vascular Disease Mortality in Texas. *Am. J. Clin. Nutr.* 31:1188-1197.

298. The Metropolitan Water District of Southern California. 1979. *Results of Bottled Water Analysis.* March.

299. Van Lanker, J.L. 1977. Smoking and Disease. In National Institute on Drug Abuse. pp.230-283.

300. Lentz, P.E. and DiLuzio, N.R. 1974. Peroxidation of Lipids in Alveolar Macrophages. *Arch. Environ. Health* 128:279-282.

301. Wynder, E.L. 1979. Interrelationships of Smoking to Other Variables and Preventive Approaches. In *Research on Smoking Behavior.* eds. M.E. Jarvik, J. Cullen et al. National Institute on Drug Abuse. pp. 67-94.

302. Naeye, R.L. and Truong, L.D. 1977. Effects of Cigarette Smoking on Intramyocardial Arteries and Arterioles in Man. *A.J.C.P.* 68(4):493-498.

303. Daniell, H.W. 1972. Osteoporosis and Smoking. *JAMA* 221:509.

304. Sarin, C.L., Austin, J.C. et al. 1974. Effects of Smoking on Digital Blood-Flow Velocity. *JAMA* 229(10):1327.

305. Jarvik, M.E. 1977. Biological Factors Underlying the Smoking Habit. In *Research on Smoking Behavior*. Nat'l. Institute on Drug Abuse. pp. 122-135.

306. Resnik, R., Brink, G.W. et al. 1979. Catecholamine-Mediated Reduction in Uterine Blood Flow After Nicotine Infusion in the Pregnant Ewe. *J. Clin. Invest.* 63(6):1133-1136.

307. American Cancer Society. 1979. *Cancer Prevention Study: A Report on Twenty Years of Progress.*

308. Simko, V. and Kelley, R.E. 1979. Effect of Chronic Intermittent Exercise on Biliary Lipids, Plasma Lecithin, Acyltransferase and Red Blood Cell Lipids in Rats. *Am. J. Clin. Nutr.* 32(7):1376-1380.

309. Ismail, A.H. and Trachtman, L.E. 1973. Jogging the Imagination. *Psychology Today* 6(10):78-82.

310. Black, J., Chesler, G.B. et al. 1979. The Painlessness of the Long Distance Runner. *Medical J. of Australia* June 2, p. 522-3.

311. Aloia, J.F., Cohen, S.H. et al. 1978. Skeletal Mass and Body Composition in Marathon Runners. *Metabolism* 27(12):1793-1796.

312. Zinman, B., Vranik, M. et al. 1979. The Role of Insulin in the Metabolic Response to Exercise in Diabetic Man. *Diabetes* 28(Suppl. 1):76-81.

313. Katch, V.L., Martin, R. et al. 1979. Effects of Exercise Intensity on Food Consumption in the Male Rat. *Am. J. Clin. Nutr.* 32:1401-1407.

314. Ahlborg, G. and Felig, P. 1977. Substrate Utilization During Prolonged Exercise Preceded by Ingestion of Glucose. *Am. J. Physiol.* 233:E188-E194.

315. Soman, V.R., Koivisto, V.A. et al. 1979. Increased Insulin Sensitivity and Insulin Binding After Physical Training. *JAMA* 301(22):1200-1204.

316. Vranic, M., Horvath, S. et al. 1979. Exercise and Diabetes: An Overview. *Diabetes* 28(1):107-110.

317. Saltin, B., Lingarde, M. et al. 1979. Physical Training and Glucose Tolerance in Middle-aged Men With Chemical Diabetes. *Diabetes* 28(Suppl. 1):30-32.

318. Wahren, J. 1979. Glucose Turnover During Exercise in Healthy Man and Patients with Diabetes Mellitus. *Diabetes* 28(Suppl. 1)82-88.

319. Emiola, L. and O'Shea, J.P. 1978. Effects of Physical Activity and Nutrition on Bone Density Measured by Radiographic Techniques. *Nutrition Reports International* 17(6):669-681.